Praise for *Newborn 101*

"*Newborn 101* may look like your typical guide to pregnancy and baby care, but it's not. It's better, filled with well-researched tips from a professional who is also an experienced mom, tips that you probably have not heard before. . . . A must-have!" —*baystateparent* magazine

"*Newborn 101* is chock-full of the kind of practical and helpful information that only an insider like Carole Arsenault would know. This book contains everything a couple needs to prepare for the adventure of labor and birth." —**CHRISTIANE NORTHRUP, MD**, author of *Women's Bodies, Women's Wisdom*

"The stack of books available on breastfeeding, pregnancy, and postpartum can be overwhelming. Carole Arsenault covers all these topics and then some—including prenatal exercise and nutrition, choosing a pediatrician, raising a 'green baby,' and more. The Q&A format and highlighted baby care tips make this book fun to read and easy to use. I'm making *Newborn 101* my number one must-read book for new parents!" —**TAMARA JESSIMAN**, Certified Nurse Midwife, Mount Auburn Hospital

"Birthing and caring for a baby is a transformative experience, and *Newborn 101* helps new families make their way with confidence. It's highly readable—and packed with insightful and helpful Q&As, lists, and tips." —**JOHANNA MYERS MCCHESNEY**, cofounder and CEO of Isis Parenting, Inc.

Testimonials

"As a pediatrician, I figured having a baby would be a breeze. When I found out I was having twins, I was even more excited. However, the wealth of knowledge gained from studying pediatrics did not fully prepare me for the first few months as a new parent. *Newborn 101* has been a valuable resource to our family: It's easy to read, has real-life tips on how to care for your baby, and gives practical advice on how to care for yourself during this difficult period. Most importantly to me as a practicing pediatrician, it's up-to-date and evidence based. As a pediatrician *and* a mom of twins, I truly believe this is a must-read book and I recommend it to all my new parents. You will not be disappointed!"

—**CARRIE D. STUCKEN, MD, FAAP,** pediatrician, Pediatric Partners, and affiliate assistant professor of pediatrics, Florida Atlantic University Charles E. Schmidt School of Medicine

"Newborns don't come with manuals! We get detailed instruction books when we buy a car, a cell phone and even a toaster, but not when we bring home a precious child. *Newborn 101* is the manual we have been waiting for! This book guides new parents through the amazing yet often overwhelming experience of caring for a newborn. I only wish I had a copy when I had my first child!"

—**PAULA J. MCEVOY, MD,** pediatrician (and mother of four)

"*Newborn 101* remains an excellent resource for both new and experienced parents. It has been updated to include the latest information available, and Carole Arsenault provides enjoyable, easy-to-read, and nonjudgmental tips on caring for your baby!"

—**CATHY CAILLOUETTE,** pediatric nurse practitioner

NEWBORN
• 101 •

*Secrets from Expert Nurses on Preparing
and Caring for Your Baby at Home*

UPDATED AND EXPANDED SECOND EDITION

Carole Kramer Arsenault, RN, IBCLC

Foreword by William Camann, MD
Director of Obstetric Anesthesiology, Brigham and Women's Hospital

THE EXPERIMENT
NEW YORK

Library of Congress Cataloging-in-Publication Data

Names: Arsenault, Carole Kramer, author.
Title: Newborn 101 : secrets from expert nurses on preparing and caring for
   your baby at home / Carole Kramer Arsenault, RN, IBCLC.
Other titles: Baby nurse bible
Description: Updated and expanded second edition. | New York : The
   Experiment, LLC, 2017. | Revision of: Baby nurse bible. c2011. | Includes
   index.
Identifiers: LCCN 2017008398 (print) | LCCN 2017010021 (ebook) | ISBN
   9781615193851 (pbk.) | ISBN 9781615193868 (ebook)
Subjects: LCSH: Infants--Care--Handbooks, manuals, etc. | Infants--Health and
   hygiene.
Classification: LCC RJ61 .A685 2017 (print) | LCC RJ61 (ebook) | DDC
   618.92/01--dc23
LC record available at https://lccn.loc.gov/2017008398

ISBN 978-1-61519-385-1
Ebook ISBN 978-1-61519-386-8
First Edition ISBN 978-1-61519-014-0

Cover design by Sarah Schneider
Cover photograph © Simarik | iStock
Author photograph © Hughes Photography

Text design by Pauline Neuwirth,
   Neuwirth & Associates, Inc.
Additional text design by Sarah Schneider

Manufactured in the United States of America
Distributed by Workman Publishing Company
Distributed simultaneously in Canada by Thomas Allen & Son Ltd.

First printing May 2017
10 9 8 7 6 5 4 3 2 1

This book is dedicated to my three children,
Alex, Cam, and Caroline, and to my niece Emmie.

*"A hundred years from now it will not matter
what my bank account was, the sort of house I lived in,
or the kind of car I drove . . . but the world may be different
because I was important in the life of a child."*
—FOREST E. WITCRAFT

Contents

Foreword

by William Camann, MD

Patients encounter a wide variety of personnel when they go to a hospital or seek medical care. Physicians, nurses, various specialists, technicians, receptionists, security officers, parking attendants, and others will all be part of the experience. Each may lay claim to some particular knowledge or insight about what really goes on in the world of health care. And each indeed does have a particular perspective with which they see the medical world. Opinions vary as to who has the clearest view—but it's my belief that there is no greater vantage point than that of the nurse.

Thus, it gives me great pleasure to write this foreword to *Newborn 101: Secrets from Expert Nurses on Preparing and Caring for Your Baby at Home*. Pregnancy and childbirth is something most parents experience only once or just a few times. The experience can be daunting, challenging, and overwhelming, as new parents are often intimidated by their newborns and struggle over even the smallest decisions about their care. Yet professionals who work in the maternity environment see new parents on a daily basis. They know the joys, the problems, the concerns, and most importantly, the questions that are asked over and over again by new parents. In today's technology-laden world, new parents are exposed, perhaps even overexposed, to an ever-increasing volume of information from family, friends, acquaintances, books, magazines, websites, social media, and other resources. Moreover, in an environment of such information overload, many of the resources are presented with specific agendas, causing even more confusion. "Just who can I trust?!" is a common concern among new parents, and, for that matter, all health-care consumers. And, when all is said and done, it is often nurses who field the majority of questions from patients.

The critical role of nurses in health care is well recognized by many, including physicians. As doctors, we speak with and examine our patients, look at laboratory test results, X-rays, scans, and monitors, and seek out the advice of consultants. Yet any doctor will admit that there is no more valuable information than the nurse's answer to a simple question such as "How is the patient doing today?"

I can think of no more uniquely qualified nurse than Carole Arsenault to help guide first-time parents through the information overload that defines new parenthood. I know Carole from almost two decades of working as colleagues in the labor and delivery unit at Boston's Brigham and Women's Hospital, one of the busiest maternity hospitals in the country. In addition to her extensive hands-on experience with women giving birth, Carole also has years of experience as the founder of Boston Baby Nurses, a Boston-area agency that helps parents though all aspects of preparing and caring for their newborns, providing education, lactation support, home care, and more. Carole and her team of skilled, seasoned nurses have seen it all, and *Newborn 101* is a compilation of their knowledge. This book covers how to prepare your home before the birth, what will happen in the hospital during and immediately after birth, and how to adjust during the first months of life with your new baby. Written in a practical, easy-to-follow, and conversational tone, this useful manual is a must-read for new parents.

WILLIAM CAMANN, MD, is the director of obstetric anesthesiology at Brigham and Women's Hospital in Boston and the coauthor of *Easy Labor: Every Woman's Guide to Choosing Less Pain and More Joy During Childbirth.* Dr. Camann is also an associate professor of anesthesia at Harvard Medical School and former president of the Society for Obstetric Anesthesia and Perinatology. An internationally recognized authority on obstetric anesthesia and pain control during childbirth, Dr. Camann has appeared on the *Today* show with Katie Couric, *ABC World News Tonight,* and *Good Morning America.* He lives in Boston.

Introduction

I can still feel the excitement and anxiousness my husband and I experienced leading up to and after the birth of each of our three babies—especially our first. Birthing and taking care of a newborn was unknown territory to us, and that emotion-filled time of love and learning was amazing. And as a nurse, lactation consultant, and parent educator to hundreds of families over the past decade, I've been privileged to guide moms and dads in their own emotional and educational transitions into the incredible, albeit challenging, world of parenthood.

The experience of modern parents-to-be is very different than it once was because there's so much information at your disposal. Just to learn the basics of birth or newborn care, you now have to sort through a mass of often outdated information and decide which pregnancy, birth, and infant products and resources are best and most trustworthy. Keeping this challenge—and you—in mind, I wrote *Newborn 101*. Applying my professional experience and, just as important, the wisdom that comes only from a mom who has been there, *Newborn 101* elaborates on key information and methods you need to make this sometimes overwhelming phase simultaneously one of utter joy. I invite you to discover the answers to all of your questions about the months leading up to the birth of your baby, the birthing process, understanding your newborn's needs, and how to soothe and care for your infant (and yourself!) during the first three months.

Every step in this journey you're on is an important one—something I've come to know through each of my professional experiences. I started out by practicing for many years as a labor and delivery nurse at Brigham and Women's Hospital in Boston, where I learned, day after day, that each mom is unique, laboring and birthing in her own way. Your birth experience will be entirely different from your sister's, your mom's, and your best friend's. I vividly recall, early on, reassuring one particular mom in her mid-twenties as she was about to push her baby out. She had been so calm throughout labor, using her breathing techniques, but suddenly began to feel tired and panicked and decided out loud, "I can't do this." Knowing that this was a sign she was nearing the end of her labor, I quietly reassured her she could do this and that she would soon be holding her baby. Her baby was born ten minutes later. The very next day I was at the bedside of a laboring woman of similar age who opted for an epidural to ease the feeling of contractions. When it came time for her to push out her baby, instead of needing calm reassurance she responded to more energetic support. She really gave it her all in pushing when she heard she was being rooted for, and she also met her baby soon after.

In addition to guiding women in labor and birth at Brigham and Women's Hospital, I regularly witnessed the bonding and benefits that initial breastfeeding gave to both moms and babies, which inspired me to become a certified lactation consultant. Since then I've provided lactation consulting to new moms delivering at many of Boston's top hospitals, including Brigham and Women's, Beth Israel Deaconess, St. Elizabeth, Newton-Wellesley, Massachusetts General, and Mount Auburn. Through this work I've seen that although breastfeeding is easier for some than for others, it doesn't just come naturally for any mom or baby. It takes practice and dedication, sometimes needs intervention, and unfortunately is sometimes not possible. Realizing that there were in fact many ways I could help parents through pregnancy, labor, birth, postpartum, and the newborn period, I also began teaching parent education courses and founded Boston Baby Nurses, LLC, a Boston-based agency that provides overnight lactation and postpartum services to women and babies in their homes. I have also found ways to reach out to families by contributing health advice to the online publications bostonmamas.com and thebump.com and by consulting for the Abbott Laboratories Pediatric Advisory Committee.

I had each and every one of these patients and clients in mind when I wrote *Newborn 101*, so I could offer moms like you the same support and encouragement I have given to new Boston-area moms over the years. *Newborn 101* is my latest venture in my dedication to helping parents-to-be during this special time. It is your comprehensive pregnancy, postpartum, and newborn baby guide: here I share how to choose safe baby products, what to pack for the hospital and what to expect while there, and details about newborn care, breast- and bottle-feeding, soothing, sleeping, and infant development. In addition to the up-to-date baby information, I provide you with the following essential resources to aid you along the way:

- To save you time in preparation for baby, I include lists outlining essentials to pack for the hospital. I present the must-have baby items and save you money by identifying those you can easily do without. I also provide advice on how to create a safe, nontoxic, "green" home for your baby.

- To help you settle in on your first few hectic days and weeks home from the hospital and carve out time for you in the ensuing weeks and months, I offer samples of realistic, flexible daily routines to follow.

- Throughout the book, to answer many of the questions you will inevitably have in the early days of your baby's life, I use the questions I have heard asked most frequently in my years of experience working with new and expectant parents. I answer each one in depth and share with you the current information I teach to parents in childbirth education, newborn education, and breastfeeding classes and parents I work with as a baby nurse in their homes.

- To equip you with a range of knowledge for your journey into parenthood, each chapter also includes valuable baby care tips (gathered from my experience with everyday moms and dads who have all experienced this delightfully trying period).

I wrote *Newborn 101* to enable you—to help prepare you for the arrival of your baby, understand each of your newborn's needs and behaviors, and take care of yourself. Through this book, as a baby nurse and fellow mother, I hope to give you the experience, knowledge, and support that will help you transition into your new role as a parent and care for your baby with success, confidence, and happiness.

PART I

Getting Ready

Preparing for Your Baby's Arrival

Congratulations—you're expecting! So now what? While nine months may seem like an eternity, they provide much-needed time to plan and prepare for life with your new baby, because you'll be fully immersed in parenthood before you know it! And I know the idea of preparing for a newborn can be overwhelming—I hear this from new and expectant parents I work with on a daily basis—but a little organization up front can help you feel much more in control. Don't worry if you have a zillion questions, ranging from what type of diapers you should use to car seat selection and safe sleeping—every parent has these questions, whether they admit it or not. This chapter will help you get everything in order for your new arrival, breaking down a few key areas you'll want to focus on: finding a childbirth class, choosing a pediatrician, planning the nursery, and preparing for the birth. Based on experience both personal and professional, I'll give you the inside scoop—like which baby items you can do without.

Prenatal and Childbirth Education

The more you learn about the process of having a baby, the more confident you will be during labor and your first weeks at home with your newborn. I recently got a call from an obstetrician about a pregnant patient who suffered from panic attacks. She was very worried about the process of labor and birth. We set up a semi-private childbirth class, with just a few couples, and focused on the fact that birth is normal and not something to be feared, but embraced. I helped her to understand that having a baby in a hospital setting does not necessarily make it a medical event. The support and information she received in the birth class gave her the confidence she needed—she went on to have a "fabulous" labor and called to tell me that hearing all about what to expect straight from an experienced labor and delivery nurse made all the difference. That's why taking a childbirth class—or several—is a good idea.

Childbirth classes will teach you what to expect during the many stages of labor and birth and how to prepare your body and mind. The content of childbirth classes can vary, though, so it's a good idea to review class descriptions prior to enrolling. For example, if you are planning an unmedicated childbirth—one void of routine birth interventions such as Pitocin (a synthetic form of oxytocin intended to speed up labor), fetal monitoring, and pain medications including epidurals—you will want to take a class such as Lamaze or Bradley. (These classes are discussed in more detail later in this chapter.) Other classes on baby care will delve into topics such as breastfeeding and infant CPR.

Some classes are offered in a series of short sessions (usually over the course of a month or so) while others are completed in just one day. You may want to take one, two, or even more classes to feel prepared and get all of your questions answered; or you can take one general class that will touch upon several important topics from birthing to breastfeeding and baby care. This type of class may be all you need, especially if you have some prior knowledge of infant care and are already confident in your level of birth education and choices.

Q. My hospital offers many types of prenatal classes. Should I take all of them? How do I know which ones will be the most helpful to me?

A. Start by discussing the list of available classes with your health-care provider and asking for recommendations. Then do some online research of additional classes in your area, because your hospital is probably not your only resource. Local childbirth educators may offer independent or private classes, and maternity stores and baby centers may run workshops as well.

Discuss the class options with your partner as well as your health-care provider, and prioritize the birth and baby care areas in which you would like particular guidance. If you are planning or considering an unmedicated childbirth, for example, you might prefer a class that spends more time on nonmedical comfort measures and delivery methods. However, if you are certain that you want epidural anesthesia for pain relief during labor, you may want to enroll in a general birth education class, as the two classes will likely vary in price and duration.

baby care tip

One of the best ways to find a good local childbirth class is to simply ask friends and family members who have given birth in recent years. Just be sure the content of the class aligns with your and your partner's goals.

Q. I would like to prepare for an unmedicated birth. What type of class should I look for, and where?

A. Classes on unmedicated childbirth can be particularly valuable because they center on relaxation and breathing techniques, which can help your labor progress more quickly as well as reduce stress, fear, and pain during labor. Because there are various ways to prepare for an unmedicated birth, you may have to choose a method or philosophy before you choose a course. These courses usually take place over several weeks, meeting for a few hours each week. In addition to providing a thorough grounding in an unmedicated birthing method, these classes will also provide general birth education, including your options if an unmedicated birth becomes impossible for you.

While the techniques and philosophies you will learn in these classes have similarities, each method is different; so it is important to do some research, and perhaps contact the instructors of the courses that interest you, to be sure you choose the class that best aligns with your goals.

Some hospitals offer classes that focus on natural or unmedicated childbirth while others do not. Start by asking your health-care provider about the classes offered by your hospital. If it does not offer the type of class you're looking for, chances are your provider will be able to refer you to a few local resources. If not, simply conduct an Internet search for a class that will prepare you for an unmedicated birth.

baby care tip

If you're interested in having an unmedicated birth, along with asking your health-care provider about available classes, be sure to ask about hospital philosophy, policies, and statistics on unmedicated birthing. For example, if you want to have a water birth, be sure to find out if they have tubs available and the means to facilitate your goals and needs.

TYPES OF CHILDBIRTH CLASSES

Lamaze—Perhaps still best known for patterned breathing (which is actually no longer the focus of these classes), Lamaze is now a philosophy promoting birth as a natural, healthy event. It informs parents about normal labor and birth, relaxation techniques, labor positions and support, and birth-related medical procedures to be aware of.

Bradley Method—Through a twelve-class series focused on unmedicated childbirth, this method details the physiology of labor and birth so that women feel empowered by, rather than fearful of, the birthing experience. It encourages the active participation of the partner or labor coach, and trains moms to take care of, tune in to, and trust their bodies.

Birthing from Within—Focuses on birth as a rite of passage and prepares parents-to-be through inner examination and creative forms of self-expression such as writing, drawing, and painting. Instructors of this course help participants identify their feelings, preconceived thoughts, or fears about birth, facilitating a healthy, open-minded experience from pregnancy to birth to postpartum.

HypnoBirthing—A natural childbirth method that uses self-hypnosis, guided imagery, and special breathing techniques to develop a conditioned relaxation response. During the five-week series, participants learn how to reach a deeply relaxed state and create positive beliefs about birthing on a subconscious level in order to experience labor calmly, confidently, and comfortably. Whether or not the techniques "work" mostly depends on what you consider a successful experience. Women who found their child's birth to be a positive one described feeling calm and unafraid regardless of whether it went exactly as planned.

baby care tip

You might make some great connections by taking a childbirth class. I made several friends in one particular class and we've kept in touch over the years. Even if it is just a holiday card, it brings back such fun memories of being pregnant.

Q. My husband and I have busy work schedules. Can we learn everything we need to know in a one-day class?

A. Weekend or one-day childbirth classes are increasingly popular because they are so convenient for working couples. The content is generally more informational and less hands-on, so techniques for relaxation and breathing may not be covered in as much depth as they would be in a longer series; check the class outline before registration to find out exactly what will be covered. Because these classes are in a condensed format that can last as long as eight hours, be sure to wear comfortable clothing, bring nutritious snacks, and take notes to keep track of details you want to remember.

baby care tip

Another great reason to take a childbirth class—even if your schedule is already crazy or it's your second pregnancy—is that it will help you and your partner feel more connected with each other and your new baby.

Q. I feel uncomfortable going to a childbirth class because I am single and would be going to class alone. I plan to have a friend with me for my labor, but does she need to come to these classes with me? What if she can't?

A. It is important to note that not all participants in childbirth classes are couples. It's perfectly all right for you to attend with your spouse, partner, friend, mother, sister, or doula—whomever you want to support you during the pregnancy and birth. Some women attend by themselves whether they are single or not, if their partner or support person is unable to be there with them. Speak to the childbirth educator before the class starts to let her know your concerns; she can answer your questions and make suggestions to help ensure that you feel comfortable and get the most out of the class. If you have a friend or family member who will be helping you during labor, I do recommend that they try to be present at the childbirth class so that they will be better prepared on the big day. If they simply can't be available for the class, tell them what you learned and ask them to practice the key techniques with you. Share your class materials and handouts to help them prepare. Remember that their main role is to support you emotionally. You will have professionals—doctors, midwives, nurses, and/or doulas—to help you with all other aspects of your birth.

Q. At what stage in my pregnancy should I sign up for a childbirth class?

A. I suppose it's never too early, but registering around your fourth month should give you plenty of time to get into the class that works best for you. You'll want to take the classes around weeks 28 to 30 so you have time to absorb the information, yet have it fresh in your mind close to your delivery date. This will also give you time to practice and master your relaxation techniques—and decrease the odds that you miss something by going into labor before the class ends! If you're expecting twins, take your class between weeks 20 and 28, as the chance for prematurity is much greater in these pregnancies.

Ultimately, there are a lot of advantages to enrolling yourself in one or two prenatal classes: you will expand your knowledge about the birthing process, define the important roles that you and your birth partner will take during labor, learn effective relaxation techniques to help make your birthing experience a positive one, and learn the basics of newborn care so that things like your baby's first tar-like bowel movements or his irregular—to say the least—sleep patterns won't come as a complete surprise! As an added bonus, you will meet other expecting parents from your area and may begin forming a support network for yourself, not to mention a future playgroup for the kids-to-be.

Choosing a Pediatrician

Once you have arranged your childbirth preparation, you need to spend some time researching and choosing a pediatrician for your baby. This can be a time-consuming process, but it is worth the effort to find a physician you are comfortable with. Some physicians may be more open than others about potential issues such as bottle-feeding, circumcision, immunizations, or introduction of solid foods. Also, if you plan on breastfeeding, you will want to have a supportive pediatrician available for any necessary assistance after your baby is born. Start by asking family, friends, and your health-care provider for pediatrician referrals. Once you have a list, set up in-person or phone appointments to speak with each doctor. Each provider you meet will vary in professional background and care style, so to help you find the pediatrician that best suits your family write down any questions you might have and bring them to each interview. Some pediatric practices offer an open house that helps parents learn about the office, which can be extremely helpful as well.

KEY QUESTIONS TO ASK PROSPECTIVE PEDIATRICIANS

- What are the office hours for your practice, including after-hours and weekend care?
- How does the group practice operate? Will I be talking with a doctor when I call with a question?
- What is the pediatrician's hospital affiliation?
- Does your office have breastfeeding support, including the services of a certified lactation consultant?

- What is your immunization philosophy and schedule?
- What is the range of experience of the doctors in the practice?

Be sure to take note of the experience levels of the pediatricians in a particular practice. It's perfectly all right if a pediatrician is on the newer side, but it's important that he or she can consult with more-experienced doctors on a regular basis. This will ensure that all of your family's needs are met with the highest possible standards. Another important consideration is the location of the office. Having a doctor's office close to home is very convenient, especially during the first few newborn checkups in your postpartum haze and, later, when you'll prefer minimal car time for your sick toddler!

All that said, don't agonize too much about whether or not you are choosing the perfect pediatrician. If things don't work out for whatever reason, you can always switch to another one.

Planning the Nursery: Must-Have Baby Gear

Preparing your nursery will likely be one of the most enjoyable parts of your pregnancy. Since your baby will be spending a lot of time in his or her room, put some thought into the items that you purchase for that space. A good time to start this project—and it can be quite a project—is during the middle of your pregnancy, around week 20, when you've left the discomforts and concerns of the first trimester behind and have more energy. But while buying for baby may sound exciting at first, the in-store or online experience can prove overwhelming for even the most seasoned shopper. The "must-have" lists you will inevitably come across at baby stores do not necessarily represent things you actually must have to prepare for your baby's arrival. And, because adding that extra little member to your family can be expensive, it's important to make wise purchasing decisions— yes, you need a crib, but you can do without the wipe warmer!

All baby equipment should conform to the highest possible safety standards. While it may seem sentimental to have your great grandmother's bassinet, it was probably not constructed with safety in mind. Safety, the most important issue when considering baby equipment and gear, will be discussed in depth in the next chapter.

A Safe Place to Sleep

Nothing is more important than your infant's safety during sleep (and believe me, knowing your baby is sleeping safely will help you sleep more soundly!). Therefore an obvious "must-have" is a safe crib or other sleeping place. While sleeping arrangements for your baby will alter as she grows and your family's needs change, you'll need to start somewhere. Here are some options for your baby's bed.

CRIB

Invest in a quality crib. Whether you choose a decorative colonial, an elegant sleigh, or a basic Mission-style crib, take the time to make certain it conforms to all official consumer product safety standards. In addition to checking the manufacturer's product information, you may want to spend some time on consumerreports.org (which charges a low monthly subscription fee). This will be extremely helpful in selecting the right crib: *Consumer Reports* provides unbiased consumer reviews on cribs at every price point, covering construction, durability, and safety (nothing beats finding out about a company's long recall history before you buy).

Crib mattresses are usually sold separately, so be sure to purchase one that fits tightly enough into the crib frame that there is no space between the rails or slats of the crib and the mattress. You can choose either a foam or an innerspring mattress, but it should be firm either way. If you want to go with a foam mattress look for high-density foam, as the denser it is, the more support and firmness the mattress has. If you opt for an innerspring mattress, look for one with a coil count of at least 150 for adequate firmness. Innerspring mattresses are usually more expensive, but they keep their shape and last longer than foam mattresses.

baby care tip

Check the dimensions of crib bedding—sheets should fit tightly around the mattress. Wash all linens in a hypoallergenic detergent free of dyes and perfumes, and don't be afraid to return them to the store if they shrink!

Q. I registered for bedding and the set includes a crib bumper. Is it OK to use?

A. The AAP states that bumper pads should not be used in cribs. There is no evidence that bumpers prevent injuries, and there is a potential risk of suffocation, strangulation, or entrapment.

CO-SLEEPER

If you're interested in sleeping as close to your baby as possible without sharing a bed, the co-sleeper is a must-have. This option will give both you and your baby that close family-bed feeling without the risks associated with sharing an adult bed. The co-sleeper actually attaches to and can be adjusted to the same height as your bed. This makes nighttime feeding and cuddling much easier, too.

BASSINET

Although it's perfectly fine for newborns to sleep in a crib, you may feel more comfortable, especially during those early weeks, with your sleeping baby nearby. Bassinets tend to be smaller and more portable than traditional cribs and can be conveniently moved to different areas of your home so that you're always just an arm's reach away. Keep in mind, however, that because of the bassinet's small size, many infants outgrow them by the time they are two or three months old.

baby care tip

If you decide to purchase a bassinet, consider a portable crib, commonly known as a Pack 'n Play after the popular models made by Graco. A portable crib can be used as a bassinet but is slightly bigger, so that as your baby grows it can still be a functional piece of baby gear. Pack 'n Plays are easy to transport, fold, and store, and can be used as a sleeping area when traveling. Some even come with a platform attachment for diapering (perfect for midnight changes!), a vibration attachment with additional soothing sounds, and a musical mobile for play.

Travel Gear: Car Seats and Strollers

Ensuring your baby's safety is one of the most important jobs you'll have as a new parent. From a simple walk around the corner or ride to the grocery store to a long flight or eight-hour road trip, you need to have safe travel gear that works with your lifestyle. One expectant mom in my childbirth education class lightly joked about the amount of time her husband spent scouring customer and consumer reviews about car seats. She had told him that they would simply buy the name-brand seat that "everyone" had—thinking it had to be the best and safest option or else no one would buy it. But her husband was right to spend some time finding a seat that worked with their budget and needs. Even the most trusted name brands make products with defects or poor design, so it's important to do a bit of research. That way you can be sure the items your baby will spend lots of time traveling in are both safe and comfortable.

Q. We don't believe in buying baby things until after the baby is born. Are there any items we really need to buy ahead of time?

A. You aren't alone—I have come across families who, for personal or cultural reasons, prefer not to purchase any baby supplies or equipment until after their baby is born. While your beliefs are important, it is also important that you have some basic items ready when your baby comes home from the hospital. At a minimum, you will need a safe way for your baby to get home (a car seat), a safe place for your baby to sleep, bedding, diapers, and some newborn clothing.

CAR SEAT

Purchase a new rather than a used car seat. All car seats on the U.S. market must meet government safety standards, so any new one you buy is considered safe. However, the same is not true for used car seats, as they may have been recalled or damaged in an accident, making them unsafe.

To ensure that your car seat will do its job in the event of an accident, it is imperative that you install your car seat properly around week 37 of your pregnancy. Once your car seat is installed make an appointment with a certified car seat inspector, who can usually be found at your local police or fire station. They will check your installation for safety, reinstall it for you if necessary, and give you tips on how to install it if you ever need to transfer it to another vehicle. You may have to call in advance to get an appointment; some facilities only offer this service a few times a month and spots can fill up quickly. Hospitals usually do not provide car seat inspections, so don't wait until you're ready to be discharged from the hospital to install your car seat. It's one less thing to worry about the day you take your newborn home.

Just as important as proper car seat installation is the proper use of the car seat's harness and chest clips. You'll find these in both infant and convertible car seats. Here are a few guidelines to keep in mind when it comes to securing your baby in a harness:

- Read your car seat's manual to find out exactly how the harness works.
- If you don't have to loosen the harness in order to take your child out of the seat, that is an indication that the straps are not tight enough. You should not be able to grasp any extra car seat webbing fabric atop your child's shoulder. Simply pull the strip at the bottom of the car seat to tighten.
- If you ever notice your baby's car seat straps getting twisted, correct them immediately. Again, leaving them twisted will reduce the car seat's effectiveness in a collision.

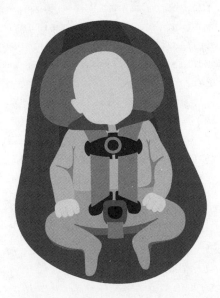

FIGURE 1-1: Baby in car seat with proper chest clip placement (aligned with baby's armpits)

- Babies should not be wearing bulky coats or snowsuits while in their car seat—as the extra fabric causes straps to be too loose and thus reduces the car seat's ability to function as it should in the event of a collision. It may seem strange in the winter, but it's best to dress your baby in layers or a light fleece while in the car seat. The car is usually warm enough anyway, and you can always have a warm blanket on hand to drape over your baby, too.

- Avoid using "bundle" type products marketed for keeping baby warm in their car seats during the winter months. *Nothing* should be placed in the car seat between your baby and the seat. A safe alternative would be a car seat cover that goes *over* the car seat.

Q. We live in the city and don't use our car much. Do we still need a car seat?

A. In the United States, a car seat is an absolute must—all fifty states have laws requiring babies to be properly restrained in a car seat when riding in any vehicle. Even if you rely entirely on public transportation, you will still need a car seat to travel in taxis, rental cars, or friends' cars. In fact, most hospitals will not discharge your baby unless you have a car seat on hand.

As with the crib, it's helpful to research *Consumer Reports*, reviews, and safety history of the various infant car seat models. There's nothing wrong with starting four to five months into your pregnancy to make sure you find the right one. Many infant car seats can be carried or attached to a stroller base, so car-free families can still get good use out of them.

baby care tip

It may seem silly, but it's helpful to practice adjusting your car seat straps on a stuffed animal or doll to familiarize yourself with proper positioning and snugness of the straps.

STROLLER

A stroller is a necessity. You'll want one for every occasion, from that much-needed walk to get some fresh air or an outing in the park to getting back into shape to easy transport at the mall and in airports. But when you need so many things from your stroller it can be tough to know which one to choose. Having dozens upon dozens of styles and brands to choose from doesn't exactly help—nor does the enormous price range from the twenty-dollar basic umbrella stroller to thousand-dollar modern design strollers that position your baby higher than traditional models to promote eye contact. So before you decide which one to start with, first ask yourself the following questions:

- How many children will be riding and what are their ages?
- What type of terrain will you be strolling on (urban streets, suburban neighborhoods, outdoor trails, indoor malls)?
- What will the stroller be used for (shopping, jogging/fitness, leisurely walks, airline travel)?
- How much room do you have to store the stroller when it's not in use?
- How often will the stroller be used—daily, weekly, occasionally?

Once you have an idea of your basic needs, do your research. The main types of strollers are universal car-seat carriers, lightweight strollers (a.k.a. "umbrella strollers"), travel systems, combo strollers, jogging strollers, and strollers for two. Ask friends and family members for recommendations and try their strollers out. Read about different brands online, including customer reviews of each product. Try different strollers before you buy one and evaluate warrantees and return policies—look for a 100 percent satisfaction guarantee.

Often stroller manufacturers put limitations on discounts, making it hard to get a great deal. One way to get around this is to buy an older model that's being phased out—it may not have some of the features of the new model, but it can still be a wonderful stroller.

STROLLER TYPES:
PROS AND CONS

Universal Infant Car Seat Carriers (Fig. 1-2(a))

These metal frames accommodate infant car seats. When you clip a car seat into the frame, it becomes a stroller.

▶ **PROS**

- You can move your baby from car to stroller without disturbing her
- Lightweight, convenient, folds flat
- Inexpensive
- Come with a large basket and often has cup and key holders
- Easy to open and close, often with one hand

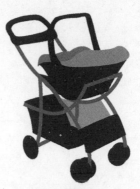

FIG. 1-2(a)

▶ **CONS**

- Can only be used while the baby is small enough for an infant car seat
- Not appropriate for rough terrain
- Not appropriate for jogging

Travel Systems (Fig. 1-2(b))

These combine a stroller and an infant car seat in one unit. Until your baby is big enough to sit upright in the stroller seat, you can attach the infant car seat instead.

▶ **PROS**

- Sturdy and versatile
- Comfortable for the baby or toddler

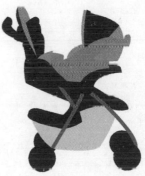

FIG. 1-2(b)

- You can move your baby from car to stroller without disturbing her
- Car seat and stroller are often sold together, by the same manufacturer
- Come with features such as a large storage basket, cup holder, and tray

▶ **CONS**

- Can be large, heavy, and a bit clumsy to maneuver in small spaces

- Sometimes difficult to fold
- Often take up a large amount of storage space
- Not appropriate for rough terrain

Lightweight Strollers (Fig. 1-2(c))

Sometimes grouped with "umbrella strollers," so named because of their curved handles and the easy way they fold up. Lightweight strollers have come a long way, and often have some of the desirable features of full-size strollers.

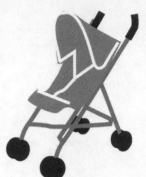

FIG. 1-2(c)

▶ **PROS**

- Generally great for quick trips
- Fold up quickly and lay flat
- Typically weigh sixteen pounds or less
- Relatively inexpensive
- Often designed so toddlers can get themselves in and out with ease

▶ **CONS**

- Often don't recline, so are not ideal for babies younger than six months
- Not always comfortable for the child
- Not as durable as heavier strollers
- Not appropriate for tough terrain

Combo Strollers (Fig. 1-2(d))

These strollers are growing fast in popularity. Combo strollers are a cross between a baby carriage and a stroller. They do not usually come with a car seat, but instead include a removable bassinet. The bassinet feature is great for young babies: because of the limited muscle strength in their necks, they sleep better in a flat position. The bassinet can also be used in the home as a portable sleeping space for the baby. As your baby grows out of the bassinet, you insert the stroller seat for your older baby and toddler.

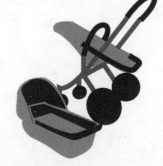

FIG. 1-2(d)

► **PROS**

- Can accommodate newborns through toddlers, up to around forty pounds
- May be the only stroller you need to buy; tend to be well constructed and will usually last through several children
- Often reversible so the baby can face you or face out
- Comfortable for your child, thanks to extra padding and sturdy frame
- Comfortable for the parents, thanks to height-adjustable handles
- Maneuver easily on city streets, beaches, and rough terrain

► **CONS**

- Tend to be expensive
- Often heavy and bulky

Jogging Strollers (Fig. 1-2(e))

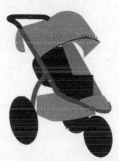

Jogging strollers encourage parents to get out and be active with their children. While they are not always convenient to fold and store, jogging strollers have become lighter and more durable. Always use the wrist strap when running with your child in this type of stroller so you do not lose control, especially when running downhill or on particularly bumpy terrain.

FIG. 1-2(e)

► **PROS**

- Large, sturdy tires
- Hand brakes
- Perform well on a variety of surfaces, including rough terrain
- Provide stability without affecting your speed
- Smooth ride for your baby, thanks to excellent shock absorption and suspension
- Can accommodate a child from six months to four or five years old

► **CONS**

- Not recommended for children under six months old unless you purchase an additional infant attachment
- Typically do not fold easily or fold flat
- Can be difficult to assemble

- Take up a fair amount of storage space
- Higher-quality models can be expensive

Strollers for Two (Fig. 1-2(f–g))

While strollers for two include double strollers and twin strollers, the two are not the same. Twin strollers typically provide similar features on both sides, such as being able to recline or accommodate infant car seats (Fig. 1-2(f)). Double strollers are often designed to hold a baby and an older child (Fig. 1-2(g)). While the features may not be ideally suited, both strollers can usually accommodate children of the same or different ages, depending on their sizes.

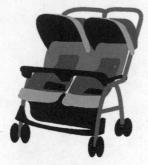

FIG. 1-2(f)

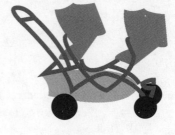

FIG. 1-2(g)

▶ **PROS**

- Great option if you're expecting multiples, are hoping to have children close in age, or want lots of space to store things while out with one baby
- Available in tandem (front-to-back) and side-to-side options (tandem strollers can fit through doorways more easily than side-to-side, but the latter can handle curbs better)
- Come in a variety of styles

▶ **CONS**

- With the exception of jogging models, these strollers can be difficult to maneuver
- Bulky and somewhat difficult to fold

Clothing (Layette)

One last area of necessities to focus on for your baby is clothes. Although I know it's tempting to buy that adorable frilly dress, cute little pair of jeans, or warm mini hoodie, it's wasted money for a newborn. All she'll need are a few basics to get you through the first few weeks—clothes that will keep her warm *and* comfortable.

Q. I keep reading about layettes. What exactly is a layette?

A. The word *layette* refers to a baby's clothing and blankets. Some pieces of a layette are more important than others, but it's a good idea to have some essential items on hand before your baby arrives. Here are my recommendations:

- Going-home-from-the-hospital outfit (cotton, one- or two-piece)
- Thin cotton cap, newborn size
- Lightweight jacket, sweater, or cardigan (2)
- Undershirts (6–12), either snap-front or Onesies-style
- Small cotton bibs (6–12)
- Sleepers (4–6), one piece cotton or fleece
- Cold-weather hat for winter, knit or fleece (1–2)
- Sun hat for summer, wide-brimmed (1–2)
- Sleep sacks (2–4)
- Socks or booties (4–8 pairs)
- Blankets in various fabrics (3–6)
- Swaddling blankets or precut swaddlers (3–6); chapter 10 will cover swaddling

baby care tip

Always dress your baby in comfortable clothing. At the newborn stage, your baby will probably not be comfortable in stiff jeans, overalls, or ruffled dresses. Stocking up on 100 percent cotton one-piece pajamas is your best bet. And because baby clothing sizes vary from brand to brand, buy them in several sizes ranging from newborn to three or even six months.

Planning the Nursery:
Nice-to-Have (Optional) Baby Gear
. . . .

Now that we've covered baby gear *essentials,* let's go over some of the optional items you may be unsure about purchasing. Some of these products can be really useful to you and your baby, but they are by no means necessary to have, so these decisions will likely come down to personal preference, budget, or the amount of space you have in your home. Think about your home and the sort of setting you'd like to create there. Where and how do you see yourself spending time with your baby during the first few months? That will help you narrow down the list of things you'd like to invest in.

Changing Table

Q. My sister-in-law does not use a changing table. She says they're a waste of space. How do I know whether or not I'll need one?

A. Whether or not to purchase a changing table depends on your personal style, available space, and budget. As you'll quickly learn, you can—and will when you're out of the house—change your baby virtually anywhere, from a grassy patch at the park to a restaurant bathroom. So if you're limited in space and budget, simply buy a small waterproof mat that can be easily placed on a couch, bed, floor, or dresser for diaper changes. If you want to create a designated changing area, here are two good options:

TRADITIONAL CHANGING TABLE
These tables are available in a wide range of price points and are typically designed as part of a set to match the rest of your baby's nursery furniture (crib, dresser, glider or rocker). A changing table gives you plenty of space to lay down your baby and store diaper-changing products, out of the little one's inevitable grasp.

DRESSER/CHANGING TABLE COMBO
If you want the convenience of a changing table but don't have space for a freestanding piece in the nursery, opt for a dresser that has a

designated changing area on top. These usually have space for diaper changing supplies as well.

baby care tip

Designate a basket or container somewhere in your home with all of your diaper-changing supplies, including diapers, wipes, and diaper rash ointment. And whether you change your baby on your bed, the sofa, or a changing table, stay close by and be wary of that first surprise roll-over!

Glider/Rocking Chair

While certainly not a necessity, a glider or rocking chair is a relaxing and comfortable place to feed and lull your baby to sleep and to soothe him—and yourself—during those fussy phases. A chair can be a good investment as it tends to get used for many years of reading and cuddling with your child, and of course for any subsequent additions to your family. Because gliders and rocking chairs don't necessarily need to be up to a specific safety standard, keep your eye out for cheap used ones online or at garage sales.

baby care tip

Whether or not you decide to buy a glider or rocking chair, make sure you have a small footstool to rest your feet on when you nurse. You can breastfeed comfortably in just about any chair as long as you have something to put your feet on for support.

Bouncy Seat

A bouncy seat is an infant chair with gentle suspension or a rocker base. There are many models to choose from. Look for one that has a secure strap-in device and good support for your baby's head and neck. Babies as young as two weeks old can safely lie in a bouncy seat as long as there is head support and the seat can be adjusted to accommodate small sizes. Many models come with a soothing vibration option—a great feature in those early months—and some come with built-in swaddling blankets for newborns. As your baby gets older the bouncy seat can be a place for play, as many seats come with an activity bar or a light-up bubbling aquarium. While a bouncy seat can be a great option when you need to put your baby down, keep in mind that some babies simply don't take to them.

Q. I registered for a bouncy seat but am not sure if my baby really needs it. What are these seats used for?

A. When you need a safe place to put your baby down and it's not yet naptime, a bouncy seat really comes in handy. You can, of course, do without one, but here are just a few ways you can use a bouncy seat to help you accomplish a few tasks around the house.

- Place the bouncy seat on the floor of the bathroom when you want to take that much-needed shower. Strap your baby in securely, and sing and talk to him throughout—he'll likely love the acoustics of your voice, the sound of water, and the warm, steamy atmosphere.

- When you need to get dinner ready or do the dishes, put the bouncy seat on the floor of the kitchen, so your baby can see you but remains a safe distance away from the stove. As you go about chopping vegetables or scrubbing pans, explain what you're doing out loud. Even if your baby can't understand each word yet, his brain is fully absorbing every experience and creating associations.

- If you work from home and need a few moments on the computer, or just need to pay some bills, place the bouncy seat on the floor next to you and make sure your baby has a toy in hand to play with. Soft Taggies—mini blankets with colorful, soft ribbons attached—or toys that crinkle or squeak are great options for infants.

High Chair

You can easily skip buying a high chair for now. Your baby will not need one for four to six months, when he begins to eat solid foods. When that time comes, even if you decide to delay introducing solid foods, your baby will enjoy sitting with you at the dinner table and being included in the action.

Q. I don't have much space in my kitchen. Do I have to purchase one of those freestanding high chairs?

A. No. While many freestanding high chairs are good because of their range of height and reclining positions (potentially allowing you to put your baby in the chair sooner and more comfortably), there are other, more compact options for bringing your baby to the table. Look for seats designed to attach to a kitchen or dining-table chair, many of which also tend to have the adjustable height, reclining settings, washable padding, and removable trays that many freestanding chairs come with. If you'd rather not have one of your dining chairs doused in baby food for a year straight, you can opt for a high chair that attaches directly to your table instead. These models are great because they don't take up any floor space, can be easily transported for use on the go, and really allow your baby to dine right at your family's level. However, your baby won't be able to recline in this type of chair, so she must be able to sit fairly upright on her own before you can use it.

Swing

Babies love motion. If your baby is fussy, a swing can be a good solution to help him relax and fall asleep. And with the many swing models available today, you can get additional features your baby may also enjoy—such as vibration, music, and an activity bar—all in one product.

Q. Since my apartment is small, I don't want to set up all of my baby equipment right away. Is the swing something I can wait to buy?

A. It's fine to wait a few weeks after your baby is born to see if this is something that you really need, especially if you have space or budget concerns. You may even have the opportunity to try one at a friend's house to see if your baby likes it.

While many swing models can accommodate a newborn using extra support, be sure to refer to the manufacturer's instructions to make sure the model is appropriate for your baby's age. Swings today come with many different features—some swing side-to-side, some move back-to-front, and others have the option of doing both. They come with soothing vibrations, music, activity bars, and mobiles. To help you select one that's right for your baby, read customer reviews online to see what other parents like—and dislike—about the each of the models.

> ## baby care tip
>
> Don't put your crying baby in a swing. Calm and relax him first, and then place him in the swing. Swings can be a safe, cozy place for your baby to spend short periods of time, but not all babies like them at first. If your baby does not like the swing the first time you try it, don't give up. Take him out, let him calm down, and try again another time. Many babies eventually get used to and are soothed by the rocking motion of a swing; however, as with anything, some babies for whatever reason just don't.

Baby Monitor

If your house or apartment is not large and your baby will rarely be far away from you, a baby monitor is not necessary. But it can offer peace of mind regardless of your home's size, as it will allow you to see or hear your baby when you're in another room. You may find it particularly useful if and when you transition your baby from sleeping in your room to his nursery; it can also be nice when you're trying to establish a napping schedule, because you'll know what goes on when you close the door. Having a monitor during naptimes can even prove humorous, especially when your infant turns into an exploring, babbling toddler!

Audio-only baby monitors are an affordable option, and even the higher quality monitors are well priced—under $50. But these days it's *video* monitors that are most popular among parents, and prices vary widely from around $50 to $400. They offer a range of features, including voice activation to eliminate white noise, night vision, and two cameras or the option to add an additional camera down the road. Many parents like this option if they have additional children. You can also opt to get a Wi-Fi camera for your baby's room that streams live video right to your smartphone.

Bathtub

Q. Can I give my baby a bath in a regular tub or should I purchase one specifically for babies?

A. Because babies are slippery (when wet!) and tend to do a lot of squirming, it is safer and easier to use an infant tub when giving your baby a bath. This is a relatively inexpensive purchase and definitely worth it. Keep in mind that, unlike some other baby equipment, the baby bathtub does not require a lot of thought. You do not need a model with all the "bells and whistles" because a simple plastic tub will work just as well as a fancy one. You can expect to use the baby bathtub for at least three months, probably longer. Foldable tubs are easier to store, and you'll want a plug at the base to allow for easy drainage and a nonslip surface pad at the bottom to help keep your baby stabilized. Tubs with a reclining design or an infant sling can help you get the bathing job done because you don't have to hold your baby upright.

Baby Carrier

Baby carriers have been around for centuries, offering women a way to keep their babies close while going about their daily chores. "Baby-wearing" serves the same purpose for busy parents today—carrying your baby in a sling or carrier can be a lifesaver, a wonderful way to stay close to your baby and have your hands free at the same time. And avid babywearers also swear by the calming effect the closeness brings to their babies. Of course, not everyone feels comfortable placing their baby in a carrier. To avoid wasting money, check the return policy before you purchase a carrier so you can exchange it if it doesn't work for you and your baby.

Q. There are so many different types of slings and baby carriers in the stores. How do I know which one is right for us?

A. The most important thing is comfort and safety, for both you and your baby, so you'll want to see if you can try them on in a store to feel what works best for you. Look for carriers that are comfortable, washable, easy to use, and sewn with well-finished seams. Here are a few basic types:

Front carrier—These carriers are made of thick cotton on a padded structure with adjustable straps for various baby and wearer sizes. The baby can only be worn on the front of your body, but she can face in toward the wearer or out once she can hold her head up. Front carriers are especially useful for babies roughly one to four months old; they position your baby next to the soothing sound of your heartbeat while you do errands around the house, and then offer a stimulating outward view on family walks and outings. If you have any existing neck strain, I would not recommend using this type of carrier for a baby over fifteen pounds or so, as it tends to distribute weight in the neck area. Front carriers are often used for babies weighing eight to twenty-four pounds.

Backpack carrier—Backpack carriers are also made of cotton or canvas on a padded structure with adjustable straps for various baby and wearer sizes. They are comfortable for the wearer, particularly when carrying larger babies, as they distribute weight more evenly around the hips and back (although some newer models of front carriers are starting to do this as well). Many backpack carriers can be worn on the front, back, or side, but many don't have an outward-facing option, which can be limiting as baby gets older and more interested in the world around him. The upside is that the baby is not simply hanging, but instead wrapping his body around the wearer in a way that naturally supports the hips, pelvis, and spine. Backpack carriers can be used for newborns (with an infant insert) and children up to forty pounds.

Wrap—A wrap is essentially a very long piece of sturdy yet breathable, somewhat stretchy cotton. They come in all colors and patterns, are easy to transport, and are comfortable around both the wearer's body and the baby's. One of the biggest advantages of a wrap is that it's so versatile. Most come with booklets that demonstrate the various positions you can carry your baby in; you can even nestle your newborn right at your chest and breastfeed discreetly. And while all that wrapping and crossing of fabric looks intimidating at first, it's really very easy to get the hang of! Wraps can be used for infants and children up to thirty-five pounds.

Sling—Made of breathable, sturdy cotton, slings typically can be adjusted and secured at one shoulder of the wearer. The baby's body is then cradled within the fabric across the wearer's chest. Of note: more than one million slings were recalled in early 2010 due to a suffocation risk, so it is critical to ensure that your infant's face is never covered by any part of the carrier. Slings can be used for infants and children up to thirty-five pounds.

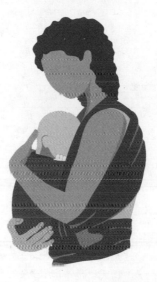

FIGURE 1-3: Woman wearing a sling with baby's head/face showing

baby care tip

To ensure your baby's safety in a sling, make sure her face is never completely covered by the fabric or smothered against your body. When wearing any type of baby carrier, double-check that all straps and material are secured according to the manufacturer's instructions before freeing your hands from your baby. Also check that any product you use for your baby is safe and has not been recalled; visit the Web site of the manufacturer or the U.S. Consumer Product Safety Commission (CPSC, cpsc.gov). If possible, register your newly purchased product with the manufacturer so they can get in touch with you if it should be recalled for any reason.

Breastfeeding Pillow

You can, of course, use regular pillows and blankets to help you get into a comfortable, supportive breastfeeding position, but breastfeeding pillows come in handy whether you end up breast- or bottle-feeding your baby. There are several different shapes and models on the market, but perhaps the most useful is a firm pillow with a flat surface that snaps or buckles around the waist, such as a Breast Friend. For newborn breastfeeding you can wrap the pillow around your waist, which helps support your arm and your baby during feeds. As your baby grows, this pillow continues to serve several purposes including a place for the baby to lounge in the early months, a chest prop for tummy time, and initial support for sitting up.

Toys

Q. I want to make sure my baby has the best toys. Can you make some recommendations about what to buy during those first few months?

A. Newborns do not need many toys. In fact, fewer is better at the very beginning. Your baby's favorite activities during the first few months will include staring at your face and listening to your voice. Baby books are a great "toy" at this age because even though your baby may not understand the words of a story, he will enjoy the sound of your voice and the snuggling.

If you decide that you want some baby toys at this stage, look for small, soft, nontoxic toys that your baby can grasp in his tiny hand when he is two or three months old. Babies also like listening to music, so a musical mobile can be helpful. Part IV will give you more specific information on appropriate activities for your newborn in the first three months.

baby care tip

Keep your receipts from both gifts and your own purchases, and keep them in a designated envelope or folder. This way, when you end up with two of the same item or feel you just don't need that potty chair at this stage and would rather have something else, you can return it for a refund or exchange it for store credit. And you'll be surprised at how many cute baby outfits you'll never get around to putting your baby in because they'll be too small before you know it! If you have a receipt, you can most likely exchange them for clothes that fit and are just as cute.

RECOMMENDED BATH AND HYGIENE SUPPLIES

In addition to the gear outlined in this chapter, here are a few smaller nursery items you should have on hand before you bring your baby home.

- Baby washcloths, softer and smaller than the adult version (6–12)
- Soft bath towel, with or without hood (2)
- Waterproof pads for the crib and changing table (4)
- Crib sheets (2–6)
- Crib mattress pads (2)
- Mild (or organic) baby soap/shampoo
- Mild (or organic) baby lotion/cream in case baby's skin is dry (particularly in the winter months)
- Baby brush and comb
- Baby nail clippers
- Emery board (should be used for the first six weeks rather than nail clippers)
- Diapers: 30-packs in Newborn size (4) or cloth diapers (36–60)
- Diaper covers for cloth diapers (6)
- Diaper pail or disposal system
- Diaper wipes, hypoallergenic (6 packages)
- Diaper-rash cream
- Cotton balls
- Nasal aspirator/bulb syringe (the hospital or birthing center might give you one)
- Nasal saline drops for baby's nose
- Digital thermometer
- Hand-sanitizing gel (optional)
- Infant massage oil (optional)

Planning the Nursery:
Unnecessary Baby Gear
·············

If you want to keep things simple in terms of baby gear, feel free to skip the following items altogether.

Diaper Disposal System

These systems can be expensive—you can always purchase a small garbage pail and use regular trash bags or grocery store bags as liners. Pails with foot-operated lids are very convenient and help to contain smells.

Wipe Warmer

Room temperature wipes are absolutely fine for your baby. Wipe warmers are rather big and bulky, and who needs another electrical cord to worry about?

Shoes

Although baby shoes look cute, they will not fit on your baby's feet comfortably, nor will they serve much purpose! Most pediatricians advise against putting shoes on a newborn's feet.

Sleep Positioner

All soft items including sleep positioners should be kept out of your baby's crib as a safety precaution. Positioners have not been recommended by the American Academy of Pediatrics and have not been proven to reduce the risk of sudden infant death syndrome (SIDS). In September 2010 both the Food and Drug Administration (FDA) and CPSC warned parents and caregivers to stop using them altogether due to suffocation hazard.

Baby Detergent

Just because a label says "baby detergent" does not mean this is necessarily the best product for your baby, though it is probably much more expensive than traditional detergent. Many of these detergents contain perfumes and dyes. All your baby needs is perfume- and dye-free detergent to protect her sensitive skin. Many stores now carry all-natural detergents.

Bottle Sterilizer

Healthy babies do not need to have their bottles continually sterilized. The best way to wash your baby's bottles is with a mild or organic dish soap and warm water. It is also fine to run them through the dishwasher once a day.

Preparing for Your Baby's Birth

Once you are all set with the necessary baby equipment and have taken a childbirth class or two, you will be in the homestretch. Have your hospital bag packed and ready to go around your 36th week of pregnancy. Even if you are planning a home birth, it's a good idea to have a bag packed in case you unexpectedly have to go to a hospital.

baby care tip

Pack as little as possible into one or two small bags—a labor bag and a postpartum bag. If you have two bags, the postpartum bag and car seat can stay in the car until after your baby is born so you don't have to make too many trips to the car upon discharge. Some hospitals require that you place your baby in a car seat upon discharge and some don't; call the hospital ahead of time to ask about their policy.

Suggested Items to Pack for Labor

- Slippers or flip-flops
- Contact lens case/eyeglasses, if you need them
- Lip balm
- Toiletries (toothbrush, toothpaste, shampoo, face or body wash—anything you'll want with you to help you feel "yourself")
- Pen and paper or notebook (It's a good idea to write down any questions you have for the pediatrician, nurse, or lactation consultant. They may only be in your room for a few minutes at a time, so jot your questions down as you think of them and have a list ready.)
- Hair band or clip if you have long hair

- Contact information for pediatrician
- Cell phone and charger
- Camera
- Music or relaxation tracks
- Lotion for massage
- Entertainment (magazine, book, deck of cards, etc.)
- Nutritious snacks
- List of phone numbers or e-mails of people to notify after the birth

Suggested Items to Pack for Your Postpartum Stay

- Nightgown
- Comfortable clothes for your hospital stay, such as cotton yoga pants and T-shirts
- Nursing bra
- Going-home outfit for mom (maternity clothes)
- Going-home outfit for baby (weather-appropriate)
- Baby blanket
- 1 copy of *Newborn 101*

Q. Is there anything else I can do, in addition to packing my hospital bags, to help prepare for my baby's arrival?

A. Yes. If possible, a few weeks before your estimated due date, arrange for household help from willing relatives and friends for the period after your baby is born. Often friends and family want to help after you give birth but are not sure what to do. Be specific: you'll want help with jobs such as cooking, doing laundry, making runs to the store, cleaning, taking care of pets, taking older children on special outings, or playing with older siblings in the house. Remember, your job is to eat, sleep, and take care of your baby. Believe me, you will welcome the help! Of course, if you and your partner feel you might want to be alone with your baby during your first few days at home, communicate that possibility to friends and family, too.

Suggested Items to Stock Before the Baby Comes

- Extra meals, clearly labeled, in the freezer
- As many staple food items as space allows
- A supply of sanitary pads (not tampons)
- Household supplies such as toilet paper, paper towels, dye- and fragrance-free laundry detergent and dish soap

The items on the various lists in this chapter will help prepare you for your hospital visit, for your baby's arrival, and for your family's return home. Having everything in order for your birth and postpartum period will help smooth the transition to a time that is joyful, yet inherently unpredictable and sometimes difficult. Hormonal changes, physical pain from birth or surgery, sleep deprivation, and emotional highs and lows can affect any new mom. It is important to engage your partner in these preparations and together build a solid foundation for a comfortable recovery and enjoyable first days and weeks as a new family.

· 2 ·

....

Keeping Your
Baby Safe

....

Parents are a baby's first line of defense. While accidents are the leading cause of death for infants and children, most of these accidents can be prevented when parents and caregivers proactively consider and make adjustments to a baby's environment. In this chapter I will cover the many ways you can keep your baby safe and secure. It is never too early to start childproofing your home to make it a safer place. Although your infant will not be capable of walking into the kitchen and opening up cabinets right away, before you know it your newborn will be crawling!

Childproofing your home may not even be on your radar screen yet, and heaven knows those first few months with your baby will keep you busy, but do yourself a favor and start going through the rooms in your home now to see how you can make them safer. Many parents find that using checklists makes childproofing easier, so I provide a safety checklist for each room in your house, as well as suggestions to make sure the baby equipment you use every day is safe. Additionally, you will learn about SIDS and shaken baby syndrome. This safety information is not intended to alarm you, but it is very important that you learn the harmful effects that everyday items can potentially have on your baby.

The goal of this chapter is to empower you to create a safe environment in your home and to help you be best prepared to care for your baby safely. Keep in mind that you do not need to childproof your house all at once; work one room at a time. I'll walk with you through the rooms in your home and answer some commonly asked questions. Let's start with your baby's nursery.

The Crib
. . . .

Q. I want to choose the safest crib for my baby. What features should I look for?

A. Since the crib is such an important piece of baby equipment, you are wise to do some research before making this purchase. Look for models that conform to recent voluntary safety standards. If the crib has been certified by the American Society for Testing and Materials (ASTM) or has earned a seal of approval from the Juvenile Products Manufacturer's Association (JPMA), you can be assured that it has passed through vigorous testing and is considered safe for your baby.

Consumer agencies such as the U.S. Consumer Product Safety Commission (CPSC, cpsc.gov) and the National Safety Council (NSC, nsc.org) have developed guidelines for crib safety. Here are some specifications that every crib should meet:

- Crib slats should be no more than 2⅜ inches apart.
- The head- and footboards should have no open or cutout areas.
- The top rails, when raised, should be at least 26 inches above the mattress.
- The mattress height should be adjustable as the child grows.

Q. Is it safe to purchase a secondhand crib?

A. The Consumer Product Safety Commission strongly urges parents to inspect any crib carefully for durability and safety before use, whether it is new or secondhand. Here are some key crib safety recommendations:[1]

---

[1]   U.S. Consumer Product Safety Commission, "Defects Identified by CPSC Early Warning System Prompt Crib Warning to Parents: CPSC to Consider Rulemaking to Address Crib Defects," news release, October 21, 2008, cpsc.gov.

- Read the directions carefully to ensure proper crib assembly, use, and maintenance.
- Inspect all crib hardware once in a while to make sure parts are not loose, making the crib unstable. If a crib does not come with all of its original parts, whether large or small, do not use it.
- Drop-side cribs are not recommended because they contain several moving parts with the potential to come apart or trap body parts.
- Make sure all sides and corners of the crib form a solid structure, as loose parts can entrap a baby.
- Any necessary repairs to a crib should be made with manufacturer-approved hardware.
- The mattress should be firm and should be the same size as the crib so there are no gaps to trap a baby's arms, legs, or body.

baby care tip

Over seven million drop-side cribs have been recalled over the last several years because the sides of the crib (which move up and down to aid in putting down the baby) can malfunction, causing suffocation or strangulation.[2] If you have any questions about a particular crib, check the CPSC's Web site (cpsc.gov/).

Q. I've noticed that many baby stores sell sleep positioners. What is a sleep positioner, and should I use one in my baby's crib?

A. The FDA and CPSC warn parents and caregivers against using sleep positioners due to suffocation risk. A sleep positioner is a device *intended* to prevent a young baby from rolling over onto his tummy while in the crib or to prevent flattening of the head. Some are made of foam and look like wedges; others are made of fabric and can be adjusted with Velcro straps. Although it is important that your baby sleep on his back, many pediatricians and child safety experts

---

2   U.S. Consumer Product Safety Commission, "CPSC Issues Warning on Drop-Side Cribs," news release, May 7, 2010, cpsc.gov.

caution against putting *anything* cushioned or made of foam into the crib because these items can pose a suffocation hazard. Since newborns are not yet able to roll over from their backs to their tummies there is no need for a sleep positioner.

Q. My baby enjoys watching and listening to the mobile in her crib. At what point should I remove this toy?

A. Mobiles are one of the best-known crib accessories. During the early months, many babies spend a lot of time in their cribs looking around and watching the mobile, and listening to the music can be very entertaining. However, when your baby starts to move around and pull herself up, the mobile may become a safety hazard. The CPSC recommends that you remove the mobile when your baby starts to pull and push herself up on hands and knees.

Q. Does it matter what color or style of mobile I choose for my baby?

A. Many pediatricians and child development experts recommend bold prints in white and black motifs because infants prefer to look at high-contrast edges and patterns. Black and white patterns present the highest possible contrast and will attract your baby's eye.

Whatever style you choose, there are some common safety tips to follow. For example, mobiles should attach *securely* to the crib or ceiling (not with string, cord, or ribbons) and be placed out of the child's reach. Avoid mobiles with removable parts because they can detach, land in the crib, and become a hazard to your baby. And while handmade mobiles are trendy these days, you'll need to make sure that all pieces are secured together and attached properly so the entire mobile doesn't end up in your baby's crib.

The Changing Table
· · · · · · · · · · · ·

Q. Do I really need to strap my baby onto the changing table if I'm standing right there next to him?

A. Yes. Remember: You can never be too careful when it comes to your baby. If you turn your body just a bit or take your focus off your baby for a second, he could manage to fall off the table. Never leave your baby unattended on the changing table even if he is strapped in. Have everything you need on hand for the diaper or clothing change before you begin the process. In addition, keep all lotions and baby care products out of baby's reach but easily within yours.

baby care tip

Place a small, soft rug (sometimes called a scatter rug) beneath your crib and changing table to soften the impact if your baby accidentally falls. Scatter rugs are inexpensive and easy to clean.

The Car Seat
· · · · · · · · · · · ·

Q. When should I purchase a car seat and have it installed in my car?

A. As mentioned in chapter 1, one of your first jobs as a parent is to keep your baby safe in the car. It's a good idea to begin looking into car seats and safety features early in your pregnancy. Many women feel much more energized during the second trimester, so that can be a great time to start researching the different styles and options on the market. Try to have your car seat installed by a professional by the 37th week of your pregnancy or several weeks earlier if you're carrying multiples.

TYPES OF CAR SEATS

Infant-Only Car Seats

Infant-only car seats often come with two parts: the seat itself, sometimes referred to as the "bucket," and the base, which remains in the car and fastens the seat in place. For convenience, some parents choose to purchase more than one base to leave in different cars. Many infant-only car seats can also be installed directly into a car without using a base; check the manufacturer specifications before you buy a seat to see if it meets your family's needs.

Infant-only car seats come with a harness that helps properly position your baby for safety and facilitate breathing. If you decide to start with an infant-only car seat, understand that you will need to switch to a convertible car seat when your baby grows to around twenty-two pounds (approximately nine to twelve months of age), depending on the make and model of the infant seat.

▶ **PROS**
- Specially designed for newborns, an infant-only car seat provides the baby with appropriate support and proper positioning.
- These small seats can double as a baby carrier.
- Parents can comfortably move a sleeping baby without disturbing her.
- The seat can serve as a safe place for the baby to eat, rest, or rock when other options are not readily available.
- Most models can snap into a stroller frame for easy transportation.

▶ **CONS**
- Most babies outgrow these seats when they are about nine or ten months old.

Convertible Car Seats

A convertible car seat, also called an infant/toddler seat, can be used from the time your child is born until she outgrows it, at around three years old. For infants under twenty pounds and less than twelve months of age, the seat should be used rear-facing. Some seats can continue to hold children rear-facing for up to thirty-five pounds, keeping them in the safest position for a longer period of time. In the forward-facing position most convertible seats can accommodate children up to forty pounds, and more models are becoming available for children up to eighty pounds.

▶ **PROS**

- Worthwhile investment because of the extended period of time your child can be in the seat.
- If used from the time your child is born, eliminates the need to purchase an infant-only seat.
- Allows young children to be rear-facing longer than most infant seats.

▶ **CONS**

- Cannot serve double duty as an infant carrier. A sleeping infant needs to be unbuckled and disturbed when going from one place to another.
- Does not have a base and cannot easily be moved between cars.
- Not compatible with a stroller; baby must be disturbed for transfer to a stroller, which can be tricky during frequent errands and outings.
- Can be more cumbersome and difficult to install and use than an infant-only seat, depending on the model.

Infant Car Seat Beds

These car seats are designed to carry premature or very small babies weighing less than five pounds. Babies who use these seats may also have medical conditions that make it difficult for them to use a traditional infant car seat. Car seat beds help position and secure babies on their backs, sides, or belly, depending on the recommendation of the baby's pediatrician. Many hospitals rent these seats to families at the time of discharge.

LATCH INSTALLATION

Most vehicles manufactured on or after September 2002 come with a LATCH system (Lower Anchors and Tethers for Children), which allows you to anchor your car seat to your car without using the seat belts. The LATCH system also makes it easier to install the car seat right the first time. If you have an older car without a LATCH system, you can install your car seat using the car's seat belts.

Q. I've heard that the local police department will install my car seat for me. Is this true?

A. Yes, but I recommend that you first read the manufacturer's instructions and install the car seat on your own. Become familiar with the car seat and get comfortable with how it works, including how to loosen and tighten the straps and how to take the base (if you have one) in and out of the car. Once you have installed your car seat, take your car to a Child Passenger Safety Technician (CPST) for inspection, a service usually available at your local police or fire department.

Q. My sister gave me the car seat she used for her baby. Is it safe to install a secondhand car seat?

A. It depends how old the car seat is and what shape it is in. If it is in good shape, has never been involved in an automobile accident, and has never been recalled, it should be safe to use. The Juvenile Products Manufacturer's Association recommends not using a car seat if it is older than six years, is missing the manufacturer's labels, or has ever been involved in a crash. When you get a secondhand car seat from a friend or relative, you can usually find out how old it is and whether it has ever been damaged. Unfortunately, if you get the car seat from a stranger at a garage sale you may not know these important details.

Safety in Your Home: Checklists Room by Room

Using the checklists provided, take a tour of your home and assess each room and your baby equipment for potential hazards and ways to make the environment safer for your baby. It is never too early to install safety equipment or reorganize your gear; the more you do now, the less you'll have to attend to when your baby becomes active and mobile. You may find it unnerving to consider all the potential dangers in your own home, but this information is meant to inform you—not to scare or intimidate you. The more educated you are, the more effectively you can prevent accidents and injuries.

Bathroom

- Use nonskid mats in the tub and on the floor.
- Protect all electrical outlets with ground fault circuit interrupters.
- Store medicines, vitamins, cosmetics, toiletries, and cleaners well out of reach—preferably in a childproof or locked cabinet.
- Put safety latches on bathroom cabinets.
- Store electric items such as hair dryers and curling irons away from areas accessible to your baby.
- Set your hot water heater at 120°F to prevent burns.
- Empty your bathtub of any water when it's not being used to prevent accidental drowning.
- Close the toilet lid or use a protector to keep it locked.
- Keep the bathroom door closed.

Kitchen

- Do not cook while holding your infant or carrying him in an infant carrier.
- Do not carry hot liquids or food near your baby.
- Do not microwave baby bottles. Microwaves heat liquids unevenly and this can lead to hot spots that can burn your baby's mouth. Instead, warm baby bottles in a bowl of water.
- Store all cleaning supplies out of reach or in a cabinet with a safety latch.
- Keep a fire extinguisher nearby, but out of reach for your child.
- When cooking, turn pot handles inward so your baby cannot reach them.

baby care tip

Even if you have a relatively lightweight flat-screen TV—in comparison to the older, heavy, and bulky ones—be sure to secure it safely so that it cannot be tipped over. Also, carefully consider the height at which you place your TV, as the screen can break fairly easily if a child runs into it.

Living Room

- Cover sharp corners of furniture (many stores sell padded corners you can attach).
- Keep household plants out of reach (some may be poisonous if ingested).
- Make sure television sets, bookshelves, and furniture are secure and cannot tip over and fall onto your baby.
- Position the cords from blinds, drapes, and shades far out of your baby's reach.
- Use stair gates and window guards.
- Remove breakables or heavy objects from lower shelves.

baby care tip

In December 2009 more than fifty million Roman shades and roll up blinds were recalled due to safety hazards. If you have blinds or shades with long cords, go to windowcoverings.org to see if you qualify for a free retrofitting kit. Also be sure to place your baby's crib far away from any shades.

Outdoors

- Keep stairs and walkways clear of debris, including snow, ice, and wet leaves.
- Check for and clear overhangs of all icicles.
- Repair cracks or chips in stairs and walkways.
- If you have a pool, childproof the area by enclosing it with a self-closing or self-latching fence. Many even come with alarms that sound when unlatched.
- Be cautious with your pets and always supervise your baby while in the presence of any animal.

SIDS (Sudden Infant Death Syndrome)

· · · · · · · · · · · · ·

SIDS is the sudden death of an apparently healthy infant under the age of one that remains unexplained even after a complete medical evaluation. What concerns parents most is that even though researchers have learned a great deal about SIDS over the past three decades, they still do not know the cause. Despite earlier assumptions, SIDS is not caused by suffocation, vomiting, or choking. Some experts believe that SIDS happens when a baby with an underlying abnormality sleeps on his stomach. Other researchers are studying environmental factors, such as secondhand smoke, that they say may contribute to SIDS. Experts all over the world are studying the infant brain, the nervous system, sleep environments, infection, immunity, and genetics in hopes of finding some answers.

A SIDS-related study published in the June 2016 edition of the journal *Pediatrics* found that the risk of SIDS appears to increase when swaddled infants are placed on their stomachs or sides for sleep.[3] It's important to note that this study does not suggest that we stop swaddling infants all together—it actually highlights the *benefits* of infant swaddling. But it does emphasize that swaddled infants *must* be placed on their backs. Once a baby can roll (typically around four to six months) it's a good idea to switch to a sleep sack, which provides comfort and *safe* snugness. The American Academy of Pediatrics echoed this in their November 2016 response to the study, reiterating:

- The association between swaddling and SIDS remains unclear.
- The risk of SIDS is directly related to sleeping position.
- The risk is doubled for infants who are swaddled *and* found on their stomachs or sides.

Another important update to sleep safety guidelines by the AAP is that infants should sleep in the same room as their parents for at least the first six months, although a full year is recommended. According to the AAP policy statement in *Pediatrics*, "There is evidence that

---

3 A. S. Pease, P. J. Fleming, F. R. Hauck, et al., "Swaddling and the Risk of Sudden Infant Death Syndrome: A Meta-analysis," *Pediatrics* 137, no. 6 (June 2016). pediatrics.aappublications.org/content/137/6/e20153275.

sleeping in the parents' room but on a separate surface decreases the risk of SIDS by as much as 50%."[4] For more resources on SIDS, see the Appendix.

Although there is currently no way to absolutely prevent SIDS, what is encouraging is that there are many ways parents and caregivers can help reduce the risk of this syndrome. Based on risk factors that have been identified by researchers through extensive studies, the American Academy of Pediatrics Task Force on Sudden Infant Death Syndrome has compiled a list of recommendations to help reduce the risk of SIDS.[5] These include:

- "Safe to Sleep": Babies should be placed wholly on their backs by all caregivers for every sleep until age one. Do not place baby on his stomach or side to sleep.

- Use a firm mattress for your baby, covered by a tight-fitting sheet.

- Do not place any soft bedding or objects such as pillows, comforters, quilts, or stuffed animals in your baby's crib. If you are using a blanket, make sure that it's swaddled around your baby or tightly tucked into the sides of the crib away from his face. Another strategy is to use an infant sleep sack, which is designed to provide warmth without the possible risk of covering your baby's head.

- Do not smoke. Maternal smoking has emerged as a major risk factor in almost every epidemiologic study of SIDS. Secondhand smoke in the infant's environment is also a risk factor. Researchers do not know exactly how smoking affects infants during pregnancy; however, numerous studies suggest that it may influence development of the nervous system.

- Do not drink alcohol or use drugs during pregnancy or postpartum.

- Breastfeeding is associated with a lower risk of SIDS.

---

4   American Academy of Pediatrics, "SIDS and Other Sleep-Related Infant Deaths: Updated 2016 Recommendations for a Safe Infant Sleeping Environment," *Pediatrics* 138, no. 5 (November 2016). pediatrics.aappublications.org/content/138/5/e20162938.

5   American Academy of Pediatrics, "SIDS and Other Sleep-Related Infant Deaths: Expansion of Recommendations for a Safe Infant Sleeping Environment," *Pediatrics* 128, no. 5 (November 2011). pediatrics.aappublications.org/content/128/5/1030.

- Follow immunization schedule in accordance with the AAP and the Centers for Disease Control and Prevention.
- Infants should sleep in their parents' room, close to their parents' bed but on a separate surface designed for infants, ideally for the first year, but for at least the first six months. Infants should *not* share a bed with anyone else (adults or other children.) If you bring your baby into bed for feeding or cuddling, he should be placed back in a separate sleeping environment, such as a crib, bassinet, or co-sleeper when you are ready to fall back asleep.
- Consider a pacifier. Offering a pacifier at bed or naptime has been shown to reduce the risk of SIDS, although the exact reason is not known. Until evidence proves otherwise, the AAP recommends the use of a pacifier for the first year of life. The pacifier should be used when placing your baby down for sleep but does not need to be reinserted when it falls out. If your baby refuses the pacifier, he should never be forced to take it. If you are breastfeeding, you can delay the use of a pacifier for a month or until breastfeeding has been well established. It's up to you how long or how often you use the pacifier, if at all; the AAP recommendations are guidelines and every baby's needs are different.
- Do not overheat the sleep environment. It's better for your baby to be slightly on the cool side than to be overheated. SIDS researchers believe that overheating an infant may disrupt his normal neurological control of breathing and sleeping, and that the preferable sleeping environment is approximately 68 degrees Fahrenheit (or 20 degrees Celsius). A baby who was born preterm or weighing less than eight pounds may need the temperature adjusted a few degrees higher.
- Avoid using foam sleep positioning wedges. Commercial devices marketed to reduce the risk of SIDS have not in fact been proven effective.

MATERNAL RISK FACTORS FOR SIDS

- Age less than 20 at first pregnancy
- Pregnancies less than one year apart
- Late or no prenatal care
- Smoking during and/or after pregnancy
- Placental abnormalities
- Low weight gain during pregnancy
- Anemia
- Alcohol and substance abuse[6]

Q. I've heard that placing a fan in my baby's room can lower the risk of SIDS. Is this true?

A. While the verdict is still not in, recent studies seem to suggest that keeping a fan on while your baby sleeps can lower the risk of SIDS. Because the fan helps to circulate the air in the room, it may lower the risk of "rebreathing" the exhaled carbon dioxide trapped near an infant's airway, a possible risk factor for SIDS.[7]

Q. I am concerned about SIDS, and know I should make sure my baby is not too warm when he goes to sleep, but I don't want him to be cold either. How do I know whether he is warm or cold?

A. Touch your baby's tummy and back to see if he feels warm—don't rely on his hands or feet, which are generally cool to the touch. For the first few months a good rule of thumb is to dress your baby in one more layer than you are comfortable in yourself. Once your baby starts to grow and gain weight, dress him in layers according to what you would be comfortable wearing. One exception to this rule is a premature or low-birth-weight baby. These babies have less body fat and may need an extra layer to stay warm in their first few months.

---

6   American SIDS Institute, "Reducing the Risk of SIDS," sids.org/nprevent.htm (accessed May 2010).

7   K. Coleman-Phox, R. Odouli, and D. K. Li. "Use of a Fan During Sleep and the Risk of Sudden Infant Death Syndrome," *Archives of Pediatric and Adolescent Medicine* 162, no. 10 (2008): 963–68.

> ## baby care tip
>
> In addition to its other virtues, cotton can help keep your baby comfortable overnight. Cotton sleepwear allows air to circulate freely and absorbs moisture from the body, both of which help prevent overheating. Some babies will wake up if they have cold feet, so dress your baby in a one-piece outfit that covers the feet, or use a pair of socks.

Q. I put my baby down to sleep on his back, but within a few hours he ends up on his stomach. Should I keeping flipping him over onto his back?

A. Most cases of SIDS involve babies who cannot yet roll over. By the time a baby has the motor skills to roll onto his stomach, the risk of SIDS has decreased dramatically. Besides, it would be exhausting for you to monitor your baby throughout the entire night. As long as you're following all of the other recommendations, try to relax and get some sleep while your baby sleeps.

Shaken Baby Syndrome

Shaken baby syndrome is a type of inflicted brain injury that occurs when a baby is shaken by a frustrated caregiver, causing a whiplash-type effect. Because babies have weak neck muscles and large, heavy heads, shaking will make the brain bounce back and forth in the skull. This can potentially cause swelling, bruising, and bleeding, which can lead to severe brain damage or even death.

While it can be frustrating and even upsetting to listen to your baby cry, the fact is that all babies cry—it is absolutely normal. Your baby may be easy to comfort or she may cry for hours every day, no matter what you do, and listening to what may seem like nonstop crying (coupled with sleep deprivation on your part) can aggravate even the most patient parent. In cases of shaken baby syndrome, a child's crying is a common trigger for frustration that can lead parents or caregivers to respond with violence. To prevent reaching this point, you and your caregivers need strategies to cope when your baby cries inconsolably.

There are many ways to handle this frustration without harming your baby. To reiterate: It is important to understand and accept that most babies can cry for two or more hours per day. But those under the age of two weeks usually cry for a reason, which is why the first two weeks are sometimes referred to as the "babymoon" period—babies this age are usually soothed fairly quickly by food, a clean diaper, or sleep. By three weeks, however, you may notice that the crying continues even though you have met all of your baby's basic needs. Understanding how to soothe your baby during such confusing times is vital so that you can respond appropriately, effectively, and calmly. I'll discuss baby soothing techniques in more detail in Part IV (with tips on how to calm yourself as well!).

There are a lot of factors to consider when it comes to the safety of your baby, but there's no need for you to feel overwhelmed. Remember that most parents have an "accident story" to tell and their babies are just fine. We tend to think of accidents as catastrophic, but most are not. One new mom called me very upset because she walked into her room to find her baby had moved around so much in his bassinette that the blanket he was swaddled in was covering his face. The baby was breathing and was not harmed but she instantly understood the importance of securing the swaddle away from baby's face. I recommended, since her baby was capable of so much movement, that she use a ready-made swaddle cloth with Velcro that could not possibly move up over the face. I reassured her that there wasn't a safety step she had failed to take in advance, but instead that she did her job by checking on her baby and removing him from that situation—no tip or safety information can replace supervision and common sense! So what I've outlined here is simply to help you take a few precautions in your home. Follow the safety guidelines as they apply to you and your household, but don't feel like you have to go overboard. Just tune in to your baby and the atmosphere around you; you'll feel confident and relaxed if you know you've taken steps to welcome your baby into a safe and loving home.

· 3 ·

....

Making Healthy
and Green Choices
for Your Family

....

When you found out you were pregnant, you likely experienced an immediate and natural instinct to protect your baby. As your pregnancy goes on, you may find yourself thinking of more and more ways you can change or adjust your behaviors to keep you and your baby healthy. You will probably make an effort to eat healthier foods, get more exercise, and in general take better care of yourself. Maintaining a good pregnancy diet seems relatively easy—just eat healthy foods, right? But do you really know what goes into the foods that you are eating? And what about your home and work environments? Have you considered how you can make these places healthier for your family?

In this chapter, you will learn about making wise green choices for your family—finding alternatives to foods and household products that contain toxins, pollutants, and chemicals. It's not about obsessing over and eliminating *every* potential hazard from your environment, and I'm not recommending that you try to do so. You don't even have to make every change that is suggested in this chapter. What's important is that you do what feels comfortable to you. The first step is to become informed, and that's what you're doing right now. Smart choices can easily make your home (and this world, for that matter) a healthier place to live. Just take it one step at a time.

This chapter is divided into three parts: a healthy diet during pregnancy (nutrition), safe personal care products, and your home environment.

Nutrition

· · · · · · · · · · · · ·

In the womb, your baby gets his nourishment from you. Everything you take in, whether it is food, drink, or the air you breathe, gets processed and goes to your baby through the umbilical cord. That's why your diet and environment are vitally important—your baby's nutrition depends on it. The cord acts like a bridge between you and your baby, carrying oxygen, nutrients, antibodies, vitamins, and minerals, and eliminating carbon dioxide and other waste products. The umbilical cord can also protect your baby from certain viruses, bacteria, and chemicals that are sometimes found in your blood. Unfortunately, however, the latest research, including that conducted by the Environmental Working Group (EWG), has shown that the umbilical cord also transports unhealthy air, food, and water. It's one more reason we should all be concerned about what we expose our bodies to—inside and out. Let's begin by taking a look at a healthy pregnancy diet and asking how to make the best choices to benefit both you and your baby.

baby care tip

Each of these healthy snacks has about 300 calories:
- 1 cup of nonfat fruit yogurt and a medium apple
- 1 piece of whole wheat toast spread with 2 tablespoons of peanut butter
- 1 cup of chili sprinkled with ½ ounce of cheddar cheese
- 1 cup of raisin bran cereal with ½ cup nonfat milk and a small banana
- A 3-ounce chicken breast and ½ cup of sweet potatoes
- 1 whole wheat tortilla, ½ cup refried beans, ½ cup cooked broccoli, and ½ ounce of cheese

Q. I've heard that I should be "eating for two." How many extra calories do I really need?

A. Assuming you are currently consuming 1,800 to 2,000 calories per day, your body needs an extra 300 calories per day. Choose foods that are high in vitamins and nutrients, such as veggies, fruits, and nuts. In order to get all the nutrients you need, make it your goal to eat a wide variety of foods.

WHAT YOUR PREGNANT BODY NEEDS

Protein
Aids cell growth and blood production. Foods rich in protein include fish, peanuts, tofu, lean meat, poultry, and eggs.

Carbohydrates
Help to produce energy for the body. Foods high in carbohydrates include breads, cereals, rice, pasta, fruits, and vegetables. Opt for whole grain carbohydrates whenever possible.

Calcium
Helps develop strong bones and teeth. Calcium intake is very important during pregnancy, as your baby demands a high supply of it. In addition to forming your baby's healthy bones, calcium helps to conduct nerve impulses, which are vitally important for your baby's developing heart and muscles. Foods high in calcium include milk, cheese, yogurt, dark-green leafy vegetables, legumes, sardines, and salmon with bones.

Iron
Helps produce red blood cells and keeps anemia at bay. Good sources of iron include lean red meat, spinach, cereals, and iron-fortified whole grain breads.

Vitamins
Aid in bone and tooth development, help the body to use calcium, help the body form red blood cells, and act as an antioxidant—just to name a few functions. Here are the key vitamins you should consume and their sources.

- **Vitamin A:** carrots, dark leafy greens, and sweet potatoes

- **B Vitamins** (vitamin B1/thiamine, B2/riboflavin, B3/niacin, B5/pantothenic acid, B6/pyridoxine, B7/biotin, B9/folic acid, and B12/cobalamins): liver, tuna, oats, turkey, nuts, bananas, potatoes, avocados, and legumes
- **Vitamin C:** citrus fruits, broccoli, tomatoes, fortified juices, kiwis, strawberries, cantaloupe, and pineapple
- **Vitamin D:** salmon, mackerel, tuna, sardines, nonfat milk, ready-to-eat cereals, eggs, liver, and Swiss cheese

Folate and Folic Acid

Helps prevent neural tube defects that can occur during the early stages of pregnancy. Sources include fortified breakfast cereals, dark leafy vegetables such as spinach and asparagus, rice, green peas, broccoli, avocados, peanuts, lettuce, tomato juice, and orange juice.

Q. I have followed a vegan diet for the last two years. Now that I'm pregnant, is this diet healthy for my baby?

A. Yes, a vegan diet is completely healthy for you and your baby during pregnancy as long as you make sure you're eating properly. You need to consume enough protein, iron, calcium, B vitamins (B1/thiamine, B2/riboflavin, B3/niacin, B5/pantothenic acid, B6/pyridoxine, B7/biotin, B9/folic acid, and B12/cobalamins), vitamin D, and zinc, which can be tricky because many of these nutrients are more easily found in animal products than in plants. Here are a few great ways to get them from vegan sources.

Soybeans—Great source of high-quality protein, and if you eat it in the form of tofu you will also be getting calcium.

Iron—Iron-rich foods include fortified cereals, whole grains, and rice bran. Your health-care provider may recommend an iron supplement if he or she thinks you are not getting enough in your diet.

Calcium—Among vegan sources, calcium is found in fortified soymilk and other nondairy drinks as well as dark-green leafy vegetables and legumes.

Vitamin D—Found in fortified soy milk, but also outside in the sun. Get outside and soak up some sunshine for fifteen minutes a day.

baby care tip

Occasionally I see a pregnant vegan mom who is having a hard time gaining weight during pregnancy. If this is the case for you, add some healthy fats such as olive oil, nut butter, seeds, nuts, olives, and avocados, as well as dried fruit.

Organic Versus Conventional Food

Although the term "organic" on a label implies that the product is a healthy choice, this is not always the case. Most stores now have sections devoted to organic products, including produce, meat, packaged food, frozen food, and health-care products. But what does "organic" mean? What is the difference, for example, between organic fruits and vegetables and non-organic ones? As a new parent wanting to make the best choices for your baby, you'll want to understand what organic really means and when it makes sense to buy the organic versus non-organic products.

To be considered organic, produce, meat, poultry, and dairy must not be treated with antibiotics or growth hormones. In the United States, the U.S. Department of Agriculture (USDA) controls which farms are approved as organic according to the following guidelines:

> Organic food is produced by farmers who emphasize the use of renewable resources and the conservation of soil and water to enhance environmental quality for future generations. Organic meat, poultry, eggs, and dairy products come from animals that are given no antibiotics or growth hormones. Organic food is produced without using most conventional pesticides; fertilizers made with synthetic ingredients or sewage sludge; bioengineering; or ionizing radiation. Before a product can be labeled "organic," a Government-approved certifier inspects the farm where the food is grown to make sure the farmer is following all the rules necessary to meet USDA organic standards.[8]

---

8   U.S. Department of Agriculture, "Organic Production/Organic Food: Information Access Tools," nal.usda.gov/afsic/pubs/ofp/ofp.shtml; USDA Consumer Brochure, "Organic Food Standards and Labels: The Facts."

Q. I like the idea of eating organic fruits and vegetables, but they're sometimes hard to find and they're more expensive than the conventional ones. Does everything I eat have to be organic?

A. The simple answer to your question is no, not everything needs to be organic. The good news is that plenty of conventionally grown fruits and vegetables have low levels of pesticides. If you're on a budget, and many of us are, rather than buy organic, choose foods that generally have lower levels of chemicals. The FDA and USDA conducted nearly 43,000 pesticide tests on produce and came up with the top twenty best and worst foods in terms of pesticide levels. The following chart will help you choose between organic and conventional produce:

PESTICIDE LOADS IN PRODUCE

Lowest Pesticide Load	Highest Pesticide Load
Onions	Peaches
Avocado	Apples
Sweet corn	Sweet bell peppers
Pineapple	Celery
Mango	Nectarines
Asparagus	Strawberries
Sweet peas (frozen)	Cherries
Kiwi	Pears
Bananas	Grapes (imported)
Cabbage	Spinach
Broccoli	Lettuce
Papaya	Potatoes
Blueberries	Carrots
Cauliflower	Green beans
Winter squash	Hot peppers
Watermelon	Cucumbers
Sweet potatoes	Raspberries
Honeydew melon	Plums
Cantaloupe	Grapes (domestic)

Q. The thought of buying only organic food overwhelms me, but I do want to choose the safest foods to eat. What about meat and dairy?

A. You're not alone. Many people become overwhelmed when they think they need to buy 100 percent organic groceries. Just one or two simple changes in your life will be beneficial to you and your baby. In addition to buying produce with the lowest levels of pesticides, I recommend using organic beef, chicken, and milk in your diet. The meat from grass-fed, organically raised cattle and chicken tends to be the leanest and has a much higher level of omega-3 fatty acids than its conventional counterpart. Omega-3 fatty acids have many important health benefits and should be included in your diet both during and after pregnancy. For pregnant and nursing women, these acids are best known for supporting a baby's brain development.

In addition to these benefits, organic versions of these foods do not contain antibiotics or growth hormones. The concern about antibiotics in our food is that they might contribute to the development of antibiotic-resistant bacteria.

The debate about the safety of growth hormones in our milk continues. Bovine growth hormone is given to cows to help them mature faster and produce more milk; cows that are treated with it develop more health problems than cows that are not. Unless your milk is labeled "organic," it may contain this hormone. The FDA says bovine growth hormone is safe, but many consumer advocacy groups are concerned that it could be harmful to humans. This hormone is banned in Europe and Canada, and U.S. consumer groups are trying to get it banned as well. So a good place to start switching to organic food for your family is organic milk.

Q. I've made the decision to bottle-feed my baby. Should I give her organic formula?

A. The decision to buy organic is a personal one. If you already purchase organic products, then yes, you will probably be more comfortable opting for organic formula. The major difference between the organic and non-organic version is that the milk used in organic formula contains no growth hormones, pesticide residues, or antibiotics.

At this time, no one can tell you whether or not your baby will be healthier if she drinks organic formula. Consumer advocates and environmental groups are conducting research, but the verdict is not in yet. Remember that "going green" is not something that can be done overnight. Take small steps. If you would rather not buy organic formula, use one of the other suggestions in this chapter to give your baby a healthy start.

Q. What types of foods should I try to avoid or omit from my diet?

A. When discussing a healthy diet, I cannot talk about what to add without also mentioning what to remove. Cut back on processed and packaged convenience foods whenever possible. Many processed meats, such as sandwich meats and hot dogs, contain the food additive nitrate. Some experts believe that long-term ingestion of nitrates can lead to certain types of cancers, so it is best to be on the safe side and eat organic meats if you feel like using them in a sandwich. These types of meats are readily available in many grocery stores and usually cost just a little bit more than their unhealthy counterparts.

And when it comes to those inevitable pregnancy cravings, avoid unhealthy processed foods and snacks that are high in fat, sugar, and sodium—these foods are more likely to contain artificial ingredients and chemicals. Many processed foods also contain large amounts of refined sugars, which can contribute to fatigue and irritability. Instead, treat that craving to a bit of low-fat frozen yogurt, organic dark chocolate, or a piece of fresh fruit.

Q. I am totally confused. I love seafood and always thought it was so healthy but now I am hearing that I need to limit the amount I eat. What does this mean, and how much fish can I eat?

A. Fish can be an important part of a healthy diet. But while fish is high in protein and omega-3 fatty acids, it can also contain high levels of mercury and PCBs (polychlorinated biphenyls, toxic industrial compounds that, with long exposure, pose serious health risks to fetuses, babies, and children). Although the mercury in fish is usually not a problem in the general population, pregnant women and those planning to become pregnant should take special precautions. If you consume too much mercury, it will accumulate in your bloodstream and may be harmful to your unborn baby. High levels of mercury in the blood have been linked to problems with babies' developing brains and nervous systems.

So what is a safe amount of fish? The FDA states that you can safely eat 12 ounces per week of a variety of seafood. A typical serving size is 3 to 6 ounces. Choose fish and seafoods that are low in mercury, such as shrimp, flounder, scallops, crab, tuna (light canned), pollock, or catfish. The bigger and older the fish, the higher in mercury it usually it is. Avoid swordfish, shark, king mackerel, and tilefish.

Generally, it is better to eat wild fish than farm-raised fish, and recent studies suggest that farm-raised fish, especially salmon, contain higher levels of PCBs. Check the FDA's Web site (fda.gov) for the latest fish recommendations.

Q. What foods might pose health risks to my baby or to me during pregnancy?

A. To avoid ingesting harmful bacteria or viruses, there are a few foods that you should stay away from because, according to the FDA and EPA, they may pose risks during pregnancy. These include some soft cheeses, ready-to-eat meats, and raw sprouts.

Soft cheeses (feta, Brie, Camembert, Roquefort, queso blanco, or blue-veined), cold cuts, and unpasteurized milk and dairy products can cause a form of food poisoning called listeriosis. Caused by a bacterium, listeriosis is especially dangerous during pregnancy. Most people would not get sick from consuming food contaminated with listeria, but pregnant women have a weakened immune system and are therefore more prone to becoming ill. Listeriosis can make your unborn baby ill and can cause preterm labor or even neonatal infection.

Raw vegetable sprouts and fresh unpasteurized fruit and vegetable juices can also be unsafe for pregnant women because they can carry salmonella or E. coli. The FDA requires that packaged unpasteurized juices carry a label stating that they have not been pasteurized. Undercooked meat, poultry, and eggs can also increase the risk of a number of food-borne illnesses including listeriosis, *E.coli*, and salmonella.

Q. I thought I would crave pickles and ice cream, but recently I've had a craving for ice chips. Why is this?

A. Cravings are your body's way of obtaining certain vitamins and minerals that may be missing from your body. The craving of non-food substances is called pica. Some women crave ice chips; others crave chalk or even dirt. Don't panic if this happens to you—contact your health-care provider. Sometimes a few adjustments to your daily diet will help diminish these cravings.

baby care tip

Pregnant women have a variety of cravings ranging from salty foods and red meat to ice cream to fruits, and vegetables. Cravings are the body's way of getting certain vitamins or minerals or additional calories, hence the Ben and Jerry's Cherry Garcia every night before bed. Many women even crave foods they loathed before pregnancy. Listen to what your cravings might be trying to tell you.

Personal Care Products

Personal care products, such as body creams, soaps, and shampoos, are generally not tested for health and safety and are not regulated by the FDA. Unlike the food industry, these items can be called organic when they are not. In fact, many products that claim to be "all natural" may still contain harmful ingredients. The skin is the largest organ in the body, and chemicals absorbed through the skin can enter the bloodstream. Once in the bloodstream, these chemicals are distributed throughout the body. In small quantities many chemicals are relatively harmless; but they accumulate in the fatty tissues of the body, where they multiply over time, and that is when they can pose a health risk. During pregnancy, some of these harmful chemicals may pass through the placenta and reach your baby.

Trying to figure out whether a product is safe can be tricky. It is important to read the labels, but this may not always provide you with a clear-cut answer. Most of us are not familiar with all of the chemical terms listed as ingredients on personal care products; many of us cannot even pronounce these words! A good rule of thumb is to buy products that contain ingredients that you actually have heard of. Truly organic shampoos will contain just a few natural ingredients, while a chemical-based shampoo usually has a lengthy list of unpronounceable ones.

Q. Where can I learn more about the safety of personal care products?

A. A good place to learn about personal care products is the Environmental Working Group's Web site "Skin Deep" (ewg.org/skindeep). The Environmental Working Group is a nonprofit research organization based in Washington, D.C., that aims to inform the public about product ingredients that are "potentially harmful both to humans and the environment." But it's actually difficult to discern which products and ingredients are safe because the cosmetics industry is not regulated the way that, for example, food is. According to the site, "only 13 percent of the thousands of ingredients in personal care products have been reviewed for safety by the cosmetic industry's own review panel."[9]

baby care tip

Most pregnant women are very careful with the food they consume, but it is just as important to be aware of the chemicals you apply to your body through moisturizers, soaps, perfumes, and other personal care products. These chemicals are not only absorbed but also inhaled. So apply fragrance sparingly, if you must use it, and try to use mild products on your skin.

9 Environmental Working Group, "New and Improved Skin Deep Database," news release, May 21, 2007, ewg.org/enviroblog/2007/05/new-and-improved-skin-deep-database.

Home, Green Home

· · · · · · · · · · · · ·

In addition to creating a healthy environment for your baby during pregnancy, it's important to think about creating a healthy environment for the baby after he or she is born. Many studies have proven that the things we bring into our homes and into our baby's nursery can be toxic—but it doesn't take much to make your home a healthier place. In fact, just a few changes can make a big difference in the level of toxins in your home. When you are designing your baby's nursery and looking at furniture, flooring, and wall coverings, remember that high cost does not necessarily guarantee that something will be better for your baby. Two terms to be aware of when considering materials for the nursery are VOCs and PVC. Here's a breakdown of what they are, and yet another reason to read labels carefully!

Volatile organic compounds (VOCs) are gases emitted from certain solids or liquids that can cause a wide array of health issues, from short-term runny noses and headaches to long-term effects such as visual and hearing impairment and even cancer. VOC levels tend to be higher inside our homes than outside because of their concentration in products such as paint, pressed-wood furniture, cleaning products, and air fresheners.[10]

PVC (polyvinyl chloride) is what most of us know as vinyl—you know, the stuff your shower curtain and the siding on your house might be made of. What we *don't* all know is that PVC is harmful to both the body and the environment. When we are exposed to PVC at any point in its life cycle, it leaches dangerous chemicals including mercury, dioxins, and phthalates. PVC is particularly harmful to infants and unborn babies and may cause long-term health problems.[11]

---

10   U.S. Environmental Protection Agency, "Volatile Organic Compounds' Impact on Indoor Air Quality," epa.gov/indoor-air-quality-iaq/volatile-organic-compounds-impact-indoor-air-quality.

11   Center for Health, Environment and Justice, "Our Health and PVC: What's the Connection?" chej.org/pvcfactsheets/Our_Health_and_PVC.html.

Q. How can I reduce my family's exposure to VOCs?

A. Good ventilation in your home is key. Whenever you use chemicals such as paint, cleaning supplies, and aerosol products, be sure to open plenty of windows for fresh air and circulation, and limit the time your family is exposed. Whenever possible, purchase products that have low VOCs or are free of VOCs altogether; thankfully, these are becoming more and more common. The EPA also recommends following all manufacturers' directions and discarding any unused product portions instead of storing them.

Q. It seems like vinyl is everywhere. How can I avoid exposing my unborn baby and my family to PVC?

A. While you can't eliminate PVC completely from all of your surroundings, there are steps you can take. Above all, when buying items for your home and your family, check to ensure that they do not contain vinyl chloride, dioxins, or phthalates. If you ever have any questions about whether or not these materials are in a certain product, get in touch with the manufacturer or do a search online. When it comes to schools and day-care centers that your children may attend, simply ask questions of the administration and try to work with them to replace any potentially hazardous products. You have the right to protect your family from such dangerous materials!

baby care tip

Avoid buying vinyl shower curtains or shower curtain liners. A safer alternative are products made with PEVA, a chlorine-free plastic that is safer than PVC. Many large retail chain stores are selling these environmentally friendly products.

Q. We are trying to create a healthy sleeping environment for our baby. Does it matter what type of paint we use on the nursery walls?

A. Try to use paints that are labeled "all natural" or "low PVC." These paints do not have off-gassing solvents that are harmful for your baby to breathe. Many standard brands of paint now contain low VOCs in a variety of beautiful baby-soothing shades.

Q. We're on a budget and would like to buy secondhand furniture for our baby's nursery. What should we look for?

A. This is a great idea, as secondhand wood furniture is a great option for safety as well as cost. Look for solid wood pieces as opposed to those made with particleboard, and look for labels inside the piece that might certify that the finishes are nontoxic. Even very expensive pieces of baby furniture can contain harmful toxins, so a secondhand solid wood bureau is sometimes a better "green" choice than that beautiful boutique bureau you've been eyeing. But keep in mind, as mentioned in the previous chapter, that secondhand *cribs* are not always safe.

Q. We're renovating our baby's nursery and want it to be "green." What types of flooring should we choose?

A. Opt for natural flooring such as hardwood, bamboo, cork, or even prefinished floors. If possible, try to avoid wall-to-wall carpeting, as carpets can harbor mold, bacteria, and chemical residue. All new flooring should be made of Forest Stewardship Council (FSC)–certified wood, ensuring that it's environmentally friendly and formaldehyde-free.

Q. While out shopping, I've noticed large selections of organic baby clothes. I understand organic food, but does our clothing have to be organic, too?

A. No, your choice to purchase non-organic clothing will not harm your baby. Remember that organic cotton clothing means the cotton was grown without pesticides, but there is no guarantee that baby clothes marked "organic" haven't been chemically treated. So instead of buying organic, choose clothes that are comfortable for your baby. Cotton is always a very comfortable fabric for an infant. Make sure to wash all new clothes twice with a mild detergent before dressing your baby in them so you can be sure you have washed away any substances the clothes have been treated with or exposed to. Newborns have extremely sensitive skin, and it's worth the extra wash to avoid irritation.

baby care tip
Parents' Guide to Washing Baby Clothes

The first rule is to launder baby clothes at least twice before you use them. Use hot water for at least the first wash to help free the fabric of any chemical residue. Use either an organic detergent or a gentle, fragrance-free store brand. Skip the fancy brands marketed specifically for "baby," as these products not only cost more, but they usually contain fragrance and other chemicals not recommended for newborn skin. And skip fabric softeners and dryer sheets, which also contain chemicals that can be irritating to a baby's skin.

Since you and other caregivers will also come in contact with your baby's sensitive skin, it's wise for you to switch to dye- and fragrance-free detergent, too.

Q. I hear a lot about harmful plastics. How do I know which ones I should stay away from and which ones are safe? And are they recyclable?

A. Many everyday things in our homes are made with plastic. It is important that you have BPA-free plastics in your home wherever possible, particularly those that will come in contact with what you consume. BPA (Bisphenol A) is an organic compound found in many plastics, and over the last few years the FDA has warned of harmful effects of BPA on babies and even unborn children.

As for recycling, each plastic product should display an identification number from 1 to 7, usually on the bottom of the product. These numbers help us to understand which plastics are easier to recycle and are environmentally friendly and which ones are not. Plastics numbered 1, 2, 4, and 5 are generally considered safe, while plastics numbered 3, 6, and 7 should be avoided.

Q. I've heard a lot about BPA being removed from baby bottles. Should I be worried about my high chair containing this chemical?

A. Current research supports the idea that Bisphenol A's primary root of entry is through ingestion, not through contact with the skin. Bottles, cups, teething rings, and toys should be BPA-free because these items will frequently go into your baby's mouth. A high chair is not something that your baby will suck or chew on, so this should not be a primary concern. But if it is still a concern for you there are many high chair styles to choose from, including traditional wood and BPA-free plastic models, and most can be adjusted as your baby grows.

Q. I use plastic wrap and plastic food-storage containers. Are these considered safe?

A. Plastic wrap is a convenient way to cover and store foods. However, like most plastics it should not be exposed to high temperatures such as those in the microwave or it will melt onto your food. If you're concerned about splash when microwaving food, try using a raised microwave cover or paper towel to cover the food.

Plastic storage containers are inexpensive and convenient. Look at the containers you have: If they have scratches or white patches, it's time to throw them in the recycle bin. Plastic storage containers are not meant to last for a long time. Even more important, it is best not to microwave any type of plastic. When plastic heats up, it can leach into the food that is being heated. Even if a container states that it's microwaveable, it's safer to heat food on a dish or in a glass container.

Generally speaking, try to switch to glass containers for food storage. Many stores offer a wide variety of affordable sizes and shapes.

baby care tip

If you would like to be more environmentally friendly overall, try to slowly phase out the number of plastic containers in your home. Start using glass containers for cooking and storing foods. As with PVC-free products, many large retail stores have lined their kitchen departments with glass products.

Q. There are so many types of household cleaners in the stores. Does it matter what brands I buy?

A. Many cleaning supplies contain harmful chemicals that we breathe in during use, sometimes making our lungs feel tight. The easiest and most affordable way to avoid harmful chemicals in your cleaning products is to make your own all-purpose cleaner. Simply mix half a cup of vinegar, a quarter of a cup of baking soda, and the juice of one lemon into half a gallon of water.

If you're looking for an in-store product, remember that the best cleaning supplies are those that do not contain any harmful chemicals. Read the list of ingredients and try to avoid aerosols. If you can't pronounce the chemicals in the product, look for another one. Beware of some "green" cleaning supplies; some contain harmful chemicals and are only labeled "green" because they are manufactured in a so-called green building.

baby care tip

If you have to use cleaning supplies that contain toxic chemicals, make sure your baby is in another room. Open your windows for ventilation when you're done. Do not use harsh cleaning products on anything that will be going in or near your baby's mouth; use mild or organic dish soap when cleaning your baby's things.

Q. I would like to have my hair colored, but is it safe to do during pregnancy?

A. It is difficult to be sure that anything is totally safe during pregnancy because no one wants to conduct experiments with toxins on pregnant women. However, the research on hair dyes does suggest they are probably safe after the first trimester. If you are dyeing your hair at home, make sure you ventilate the room sufficiently by opening up windows. If you go to a professional salon, opt for natural hair products.

Q. Are hand sanitizers safe to use?

A. It's OK to use hand sanitizers occasionally or when soap and water are not readily available. The problem with some hand sanitizers is that they contain a chemical called triclosan. Triclosan, which is sometimes added to antibacterial products such as hand sanitizer, hand soap, body wash, socks, bath mats, and toys, is registered as a pesticide by the U.S. Environmental Protection Agency (EPA) and can be absorbed through our skin. Triclosan is also suspected to cause cancer in humans. Plain soap without antibacterial chemicals is best, so as long as you wash your hands with soap and hot water, you're getting rid of the germs.

Q. I love the smell of air fresheners and fragrant candles. Should I be concerned about breathing these products?

A. I recommend staying away from commercial air fresheners and fragrant candles as they both contain artificial scents filled with potentially toxic chemicals. Paraffin candles also emit soot, which, according to the American Lung Association, contains documented toxins that are harmful to inhale. Opt instead for natural air fresheners and organic soy and beeswax candles. Baking soda or a saucer of vinegar absorbs smells and can be placed in different areas around your home to eliminate odors. Air fresheners made from natural essential oils are a great alternative to the commercial air fresheners sold in many stores. Finally, don't forget to keep your windows open during the day for fresh air if weather permits.

baby care tip

Make your own air freshener at home by using essential oils. Essential oils are all natural, contain no harmful chemicals, and come in a variety of scents such as lavender, jasmine, pine, and eucalyptus. Combine ten drops of your favorite essential oil with two cups of water and pour it into a spray bottle. Use this mixture to eliminate odors and freshen the smell of a room. Another great way to freshen a room is to insert cloves into the peels of oranges or put the zest of a few lemons and limes into a dish.

Q. I've noticed "green" and "organic" dry-cleaners popping up all over town. Does this mean I should switch from my regular dry-cleaner to one of these?

A. Not necessarily—as with any product or service, beware of "green" claims. Many dry-cleaners call themselves green regardless of the process they use. Dry-cleaning works by using chemicals instead of water to clean clothes, and the chemicals used by traditional dry-cleaners can be harmful to humans with constant exposure. Needless to say, you want to avoid breathing them in while you're pregnant, so try not to wear clothing that needs to be dry-cleaned, and do not dry-clean anything your baby will use. Remove the wrapper from dry-cleaned clothes outside or in your garage and let your clothes air out for at least a day, preferably four or five, before wearing them.

Organic dry-cleaners are starting to pop up in more places. If you haven't seen one, look online for one in your area—try to find a Web site with information about the process they use and/or try to find reviews about the organic nature of the service.

The Scoop on Cloth Versus Disposable Diapers

The choice between cloth and disposable diapers is one that may interest, confuse, or even intimidate you. Between environmental impact, health concerns, convenience, and cost, there are many factors to consider. The guide below contains the pros and cons of each option to help you make an informed decision about which diapers to use on your baby.

CLOTH DIAPERS

There are many cloth diapering options available today. Old-fashioned pins and cloth squares are still used occasionally, but there are also a variety of convenient newer options. With some cloth diapering systems, there are several parts and accessories: the diaper, the cover, and the liner (some liners are disposable and biodegradable while others are reusable). You can rinse and then wash the diapers yourself, or you may be able to find a diaper laundering service in your area that will pick up your dirty diapers, wash them, and drop off the clean set. These services may or may not require you to rinse the diapers before pickup.

▶ **CLOTH DIAPERS PROS**

- Cloth diapers do not add to landfills
- Cloth-diapered babies tend to potty train sooner, likely because they can feel the wetness more than babies wearing disposables
- Less-frequent diaper rash, because cloth diapers don't contain chemicals and are more breathable than disposables
- The investment can take you through more than one child, or you can sell the diapers
- Can be recycled as household rags after babies are done with them
- For parents who need to know their baby's urine output, cloth makes it easier to monitor
- Opinions vary, but studies suggest that cloth diapers, washed at home and line-dried, can have the lowest environmental impact while being the most cost-effective

▶ **CLOTH DIAPERS CONS**

- Laundering diapers uses energy and water
- Babies will likely need to be changed more often in the course of a day
- If you hope to use a diaper service, they are becoming more and more difficult to find, even near larger cities
- Soiled diapers need to sit in a diaper pail until they are washed or the diaper service comes; odors can be very strong, especially after the child begins eating solid food
- Even with a diaper service, you still have to rinse the diapers, which means more hands-on time with diaper contents
- Can leak more frequently than disposable diapers, though this problem can be mitigated by experimenting and finding the right style and fit for your baby
- Inconvenient to carry home soiled diapers when you're on an outing, since you can't throw them away
- Leaks on clothing will lead to more laundry overall, which can mean higher electricity bills and additional costs for detergent
- Start-up costs are higher than with disposables, though the investment can pay off over time

DISPOSABLE DIAPERS

These diapers are designed for leak protection and convenience. Diaper sizes are broken down by age and weight. You can try several brands until you find the best match for your baby. Eco-friendly, bleach-free, and organic options are now available, usually at a premium cost.

▶ **DISPOSABLE DIAPERS PROS**

- Easy to manage, since you just throw them away
- Traveling is easier than it is with cloth
- Leak less often than cloth

▶ **DISPOSABLE DIAPERS CONS**

- More-frequent diaper rash due to the chemicals, poor breathability, and longer time spent in diapers that feel dry but are actually wet
- Most options are not biodegradable and they fill up landfills, where some estimates say they sit for 500 years
- Can get expensive (*Consumer Reports* estimates approximately $2,000 spent on diapers until your child is toilet-trained)
- Can forestall potty training because little ones cannot always tell when they're wet while wearing disposables
- Some environmental advocates suggest that the manufacturing of disposable diapers has a more significant impact on the environment than reusable diapers.

As you can see, there's a lot that goes into making healthy and green choices for your family. From choosing foods free of pesticides or hormones to finding cleaning products free of harmful chemicals, there are many steps you can take. But just because the trend toward going green has exploded and you see its messages everywhere doesn't mean you have to worry yourself sick trying to replace everything in your home. The fact is, there is no way to protect ourselves from *all* of the hazards we come across in our daily lives. You may still choose conventional products for your family and that's OK—you and your baby will be just fine. Even making just one or two changes can put your family on a healthier track overall.

PART II

Labor, Delivery, and the Postpartum Period

· 4 ·

....

The Pregnancy Homestretch

....

As the big event draws near, you may start thinking about the logistics of birth itself. What can you expect from the third trimester and the events leading up to the delivery? How will you know the difference between real and practice labor? And, of course, when it's the real thing, when should you go to the hospital? In this chapter I will give you some suggestions on how to deal with third-trimester discomforts and how to recognize signs of labor. I will also walk you through the hospital admission process and introduce you to triage and the labor room. Finally, I'll describe the birth, that wonderful moment when you first have the opportunity to meet your baby face-to-face.

Most of your pregnancy is spent adjusting to your ever-changing body and planning for your baby, but by the end of the third trimester, the focus becomes less about preparation and more about overt anticipation. You may be nervous, and the desire to finally meet your baby grows paramount. This can be a time of excitement and overwhelming emotion as well as, very often, impatience. At this time it's important to remember—just because your bags may be packed and set to go, that doesn't necessarily mean your baby is ready to arrive!

Try not to put a lot of stock in the "due date" of your baby. The due date is actually just an estimate of when your baby may be born. Some babies show up earlier than expected and some need a little more time before making their appearance. Even though the due date gets a lot of attention, it would be more accurate to describe it as an estimated due date or even a "due month"—on average, babies are born sometime within the two weeks surrounding that date. The length of a normal, healthy pregnancy ranges between 37 and 42 weeks.

By the time you hit the middle of your third trimester, you may be so tired of being pregnant that the idea of tacking on two more weeks beyond your due date seems thoroughly unappealing. However, babies develop at different rates, and a lot of that development happens right toward the end. The best thing you can do is be patient and find ways to enjoy those final weeks before your baby is born.

Some people refer to this time as a babymoon—yes, the same term used for the first quiet weeks with your newborn! But this babymoon phase is more like a honeymoon—the idea being that you spend the last weeks of your pregnancy enjoying time with your loved ones, resting, relaxing, and anticipating the birth from a place of calm and peace rather than anxiety. For example, you may enjoy taking leisurely walks. While walking outdoors—particularly in a very warm or very cold climate—may not seem relaxing, it can actually do wonders for you during this time. Continuing to go on walks throughout your third trimester will not only help you pass the time and release some of your anxious energy (which helps you truly relax when you get home), but it can also help prepare your body for labor. The movement and pressure on your pelvis can gradually increase contractions weeks before you actually go into labor, making the transition into active labor a little bit less of a shock when it arrives. Of course, you'll want to double-check with your health-care provider to make sure activity is recommended for you at that point in your pregnancy.

While the goal is relaxation, it is completely normal to find yourself preoccupied with questions and concerns about the birth—when will labor start and how will it go? Will your baby be healthy? You may feel that you yourself aren't quite ready. Conversely, you may find that you wish the time would pass more quickly so you can begin to enjoy your new baby.

By the end of the third trimester your baby will be fully formed, just waiting for the right time to make his or her entrance into the world. According to the CDC, the average birth weight for a full-term

U.S. baby, is approximately seven and a half pounds and the average length is twenty inches. Keep in mind, though, that there is a wide range of "normal" when it comes to newborn height and weight—as with most things having to do with birth.

Third Trimester Discomforts

There are many telltale signs that you are nearing the end of your pregnancy. The energy and wellness you may have felt a few months earlier will likely start to fade. The increased weight and size of your baby will be much more noticeable to you, and you may start to feel very uncomfortable. But there is no need to suffer! There are lots of things you can do to help relieve some of the most common physical discomforts felt by women in the third trimester. It also helps to remember that you are almost at the end, and soon you will hold your new baby in your arms!

Q. I had so much energy during my second trimester, but now I feel like I need a nap every afternoon. When I finally do go to bed, why is it so hard to fall and stay asleep?

A. It is common to experience periods of low energy and even exhaustion during pregnancy—usually in the first and third trimesters, but they can happen anytime. After all, you are carrying around much more weight than you are used to carrying, and your body is working overtime to care for you and your baby.

Listen to your body and rest when you can. Sometimes it can be difficult to maintain a comfortable position while sleeping. It is not unusual to find yourself flopping back and forth all night trying to take the pressure off your aching hips. Try propping yourself up in a semi-reclined position. Experiment with different pillow setups: try a pillow not only between your legs but also under your belly when lying on your side. Another thing that may improve your sleep is to finish drinking your recommended fluids a few hours before you go to bed; this might reduce wakeup trips to the bathroom. And if you can, try taking catnaps in the afternoon or early evening. Labor is a physical activity—you will want to be as relaxed and rested as possible when it is time to have your baby.

baby care tip

If you're exhausted, re-energize. If you just don't have time to take that much-needed nap, a quick way to regain a little energy is to boost your body circulation through stretching. Here are two simple yoga stretches that you can essentially do anytime, anywhere:

- From a standing position, bend your knees slightly and place your hands on them. Slowly arch your back up toward the ceiling with your head down and hold for a few seconds. Slowly bend your knees, lean forward to flatten your back, and bring your head level with it. Then slowly come up to standing, keeping your knees slightly bent. Repeat a few times.
- Get down on your hands and knees, and keep your back straight. Slowly round your spine up toward the ceiling, drop your head, and hold for a few seconds while you exhale. Then drop your belly and round your spine downward while taking a deep breath. Repeat two or three times.

Q. Why do I constantly feel like I am out of breath?

A. As you've noticed, walking up a flight of stairs—or sometimes just talking—may leave you panting. Because of the growing uterus, your diaphragm (the thin, flat muscle between your lungs and abdomen) is being pushed up out of its normal position, making it difficult to take a deep breath.

Maintaining correct posture will help you to breathe better because it creates more room for the diaphragm to work. If you're having a hard time sleeping at night because of shortness of breath, propping yourself up with pillows may help. The good news is that during the last weeks of pregnancy your baby will drop further into the pelvis, taking some pressure off the diaphragm. And remember to keep moving—exercising throughout pregnancy will improve your breath capacity. Just be careful not to overexert yourself, and be mindful of two important aspects of pregnancy exercise—a slow warm-up and a slow cool-down. Be sure to talk to your health-care provider about any exercise program you are considering, and contact him or her right away if you are ever worried about your breathing.

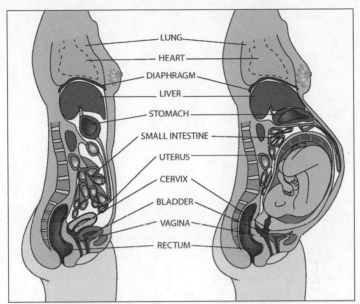

LUNG
HEART
DIAPHRAGM
LIVER
STOMACH
SMALL INTESTINE
UTERUS
CERVIX
BLADDER
VAGINA
RECTUM

FIGURE 4-1: Non-pregnant woman and pregnant woman and fetus

Q. Why are my hips and pelvis starting to get achy? Is there anything I can do to avoid this?

A. Hormones released during pregnancy cause the joints in the pelvis and hip area to relax, ultimately making room for the baby to be born more easily. It is important to maintain correct posture and use good body mechanics to avoid aches and pains as well as injury. Many women find relief by wearing a maternity belt, which can relieve back pain and pressure as your uterus grows to accommodate your developing baby. Good posture also facilitates optimal positioning of the baby and can help you avoid back labor—discomfort you may feel during labor contractions when your baby's position puts pressure on your lower back and hips.

Some basic routine stretching may help you alleviate back, hip, and pelvis pain and maintain better posture, by relaxing tight muscles. Prenatal yoga and prenatal Pilates can accomplish this and help make you aware of your body's positioning. If you're on a budget or don't have much free time to take a class, there are many great prenatal yoga and Pilates DVDs out there—that way you can squeeze in those stretches when it works for you.

Prenatal massage is another way to help your aching hips and can also reduce swelling, improve sleep, and relieve emotional stress. Be sure to see a massage therapist who is specially trained in prenatal massage. Chiropractic and acupuncture treatments also have pain-relieving and posture-improving benefits. Of course, something as easy as a warm bath and compresses can be soothing, too.

Q. I am having pain from my lower back all the way down my leg. What can I do to ease it?

A. Your baby could be resting on your sciatic nerve, which causes a lower back pain that can radiate down to the back of your legs. Move your body by walking, stretching, or doing yoga or another form of exercise. Any of these will encourage your baby to move in utero, which will eliminate the pain almost immediately. The above suggestions for lower back and hip pain are also applicable to sciatica. Try using heat or cold therapy for tightness and swelling. Alternating between different pairs of shoes throughout the week can also help.

Q. My belly is starting to get very itchy. Is there anything I can do?

A. Pregnant bellies are often itchy because the stretching and tightening of the skin results in dryness. Avoid scratching if you can, because sometimes that will make the itch worse. Keep your abdomen regularly lubricated with an anti-itch lotion or a moisturizing cream with vitamin E and cocoa butter in it. Make a habit of moisturizing as soon as you get out of the shower and before you go to bed at night.

If your itchy belly is accompanied by a rash, you could have a condition referred to as PUPPS, or pruritic urticarial papules and plaques of pregnancy. This rash commonly occurs in first-time pregnancies during the third trimester and for a few weeks after the baby is delivered. PUPPS is harmless, but the itching can be annoying and can last for up to two weeks postpartum. Anything that will help to alleviate the itch is recommended, such as oatmeal or baking soda baths. Your health-care provider may also suggest some oral medications or anti-itch creams.

baby care tip

Some women experience severe itching late in pregnancy without a rash. This could be associated with a condition called cholestasis of pregnancy, in which the normal flow of bile in the gallbladder is affected by high amounts of pregnancy hormones. This buildup of bile in the bloodstream can cause extreme itchiness. If you are experiencing this symptom, contact your health-care provider.

Q. I've been waking up in the middle of the night with cramps in my legs. Is there anything I can do to prevent or relieve the pain?

A. A leg cramp is a sudden tightening of muscles that can cause intense pain, and it's common for these spasms to occur at night. Some thoughts on why they occur include changes in blood circulation during pregnancy, stress on leg muscles carrying extra pregnancy weight, and pressure of the growing baby on the nerves and blood vessels that serve your legs.

To prevent leg cramps, stretch and massage your legs, calves, and ankles before going to bed. A warm bath before bedtime may also help to relax your muscles. When you feel a cramp, flex your toes toward your nose for a few seconds, then straighten your leg and heel and wiggle your toes. Walking for a few minutes on a cold floor when you have the cramp may provide some relief. Increase your water intake, too, since muscle spasms can be the result of dehydration.

baby care tip

To help avoid leg cramps and other aches during sleep, stretch your body out every night before you go to bed. Simply stand about one foot away from the side of your bed with your feet apart. Bend at your waist and place both hands on the bed, arms straight. Take long, slow, deep breaths. You should primarily feel the stretch in your shoulders, hips, and calf muscles.

Q. What causes the swollen veins in my legs?

A. The job of a vein is to carry blood from the extremities back to the heart. Veins are full of valves that keep the blood flowing in the right direction. During pregnancy, the growing uterus puts increased pressure on pelvic and leg veins, and those that swell are called varicose veins. They usually occur in legs and feet because these veins are the farthest from the heart—they have to work extra hard to return that blood.

To prevent varicose veins, try to elevate your legs at a right angle to your body for two to five minutes several times each day. Also, avoid long periods of sitting or standing; and when you are sitting, avoid crossing your legs. All of these things reduce circulation. If you are lying down try to elevate your feet a bit with a pillow. Wearing support hose will also help to improve the circulation in your legs. Put them on before you get out of bed in the morning, before your legs begin to swell. Walking and exercising every day improves blood flow, too.

baby care tip

If you already have noticeable veins or if they tend to run in your family, prevention is key. Start wearing support hose early in pregnancy to help keep those veins from swelling.

Q. I am 35 weeks pregnant and am developing very painful hemorrhoids. What can I do?

A. Hemorrhoids are varicose veins in the rectal area. They can cause pain, itching, and even bleeding during a bowel movement. Avoid constipation by eating foods that are high in fiber and by drinking lots of water. Sleep on your side rather than your back to take the pressure off your rectal veins, and avoid long hours of standing or sitting. Kegel exercises are a great way to increase circulation to the area (see page 85). Warm soaks in a tub will provide soothing relief; you can also try applying cold compresses or ice packs. Keep the area clean and apply witch hazel with cotton balls or an over-the-counter product that contains witch hazel several times a day.

Most likely your hemorrhoids will stick around for a few weeks after delivery. Your health-care provider will give you medications to help reduce the swelling and your postpartum nurse will most likely recommend a sitz bath (a small plastic tub designed to help you soak your bottom in warm water).

baby care tip

To help avoid or get rid of painful hemorrhoids, be sure to drink lots of water and eat plenty of high-fiber foods. Some great foods that are packed with fiber include:

Raspberries	Whole grain pasta	Almonds
Apples	Whole grain bread	Peas
Pears	Brown rice	Broccoli
Bananas	Oatmeal	Carrots
Oranges	Artichokes	

Q. Is there any way to eliminate the stretch marks on my belly?

A. Those reddish or purplish streaks are caused by stretching of the skin due to weight gain. Unfortunately there is no proven treatment for stretch marks, but over time they gradually fade. As with most things, good nutrition on the inside will help your skin's appearance on the outside, so make sure you're getting enough vitamin E and essential fatty acids. You can always check with your dermatologist about the possibility of lightening the marks with laser treatments or skin dermabrasion.

Q. My hands and feet are swollen at the end of the day. Is this normal?

A. Mild swelling due to the accumulation of fluids in the tissue is normal during this stage of your pregnancy. It is especially common in warmer weather or later in the day after sitting or standing for a long period of time. Shoes are likely to start becoming tight and you may notice that your rings are more difficult to take off.

Be active, take regular stretch breaks, and move around. Try to elevate your feet several times a day, and do ankle circles to increase circulation. If you don't already do so, sleep on your left side to help your kidneys work more efficiently. And, of course, be sure to drink at least eight glasses of water per day. It may seem strange to drink water when you're trying to reduce the swelling in your body, but staying well hydrated is important for many reasons including helping your system flush out waste. Fill a container with approximately half a gallon (or about two liters) of water and place it in the refrigerator or, if you prefer room temperature water, keep it on the kitchen counter. Drink throughout the day—this helps to ensure you are staying adequately hydrated.

baby care tip

Did you know that reducing the amount of carbohydrates you consume could help to reduce your swelling? Carbohydrates hold more water than fat and proteins. If you love bagels, bread, and pasta, try to switch to the whole grain versions. You may notice a difference in taste at first, but your taste buds will soon get used to the new flavors and they'll be a much healthier way of satisfying those carb cravings.

Put away your heels and choose comfortable flat shoes instead. Wearing support hose can also provide some relief to swollen legs. If the swelling comes on suddenly, is excessive (especially in the hands and face), or is accompanied by a headache, blurred vision, or spots in front of your eyes, call your health-care provider right away. This could signal the beginning of pregnancy-induced hypertension, which requires prompt medical attention.

Q. In the last few days I've started to leak urine every time I sneeze. Is this normal? What can I do to prevent this?

A. People tend to laugh urine leakage off as a natural consequence of pregnancy and birthing a baby. And while it *is* common, it is by no means normal. Having a baby puts an enormous amount of stress on your pelvic region, which can lead to incontinence (leaking) and other symptoms both immediately postpartum and long term, including painful sex and pelvic pain. There are steps you can take during pregnancy to help prevent this, and also exercises you can do postpartum to heal. I encourage you to ask your health-care provider to refer you to a physical therapist who specializes in pelvic health sooner rather than later.

baby care tip

Try not to get discouraged by urine leakage, but *don't* ignore it either. Many women need more than Kegels to strengthen the muscles of the perineum (the area between the rectum and urethra) after childbirth. Discuss your symptoms with your care provider, and if you're not referred to a pelvic-health specialist or given a rehabilitation plan, see someone else. Otherwise, this is something that could affect your quality of life for years and years to come.

KEGEL EXERCISES

You can do Kegels anywhere: at stoplights, while sitting at work, or as part of your regular exercise! To make sure you know how to contract your pelvic floor muscles, try to stop the flow of urine while you are going to the bathroom. If you succeed, you've done the basic move. Once you've identified these muscles, empty your bladder and sit or lie down. Then:

- Contract the pelvic floor muscles.
- Hold the contraction for three seconds and then relax for three seconds.
- Repeat ten times.
- Once you have perfected three-second muscle contractions, hold for four seconds with four-second rests.
- Work up to keeping the muscle contracted for ten seconds and then relaxing for ten seconds in-between.
- Repeat three times a day.
- Do not do Kegels while urinating—stopping and starting the flow may increase the possibility of getting a bladder infection, which pregnant women are more prone to anyway.

Q. When will I start seeing my health-care provider more than just once a month?

A. Starting in the third trimester, you will probably start seeing your provider more frequently. During the last month, your health-care provider will likely want to see you once a week. During these routine visits your health-care provider will listen to your baby's heartbeat, check your blood pressure, and evaluate your and your baby's overall well-being. Your belly may also be measured and your weight assessed to ensure healthy growth and weight gain.

You can talk to your provider about any questions or concerns you may have, but prenatal appointments can be short, so come with a list of all the things you want to go over. That way you'll be sure to remember everything you wanted to discuss.

Q. My friend hired a doula to be with her in labor. What is a doula? Do I need one?

A. Birth doulas provide physical and emotional support during labor. They are usually hired and paid by the expecting family, and fees vary depending on the doula's expertise and references (some have hundreds or thousands of labors under their belts!). More and more families are willing to pay these fees due to the positive effects doulas can have on the birthing experience. Because doulas guide moms through each contraction step by step (and help birth partners feel more involved in the process as well), many doula-supported births avoid the use of medical intervention. Doulas in no way replace the roles of health-care providers or nurses but instead serve as a valuable personal resource to families leading up to and during the birth of their babies. You certainly don't need to hire a doula in order to have a positive birth experience, but if you're hoping to achieve a specific birthing goal such as an unmedicated birth, home birth, or vaginal birth after cesarean, then hiring a doula may be a good choice for you. For more information about the role of a doula, and to find one in your area, visit the DONA International Web site (dona.org).

baby care tip

If you're interested in hiring a doula for the birth of your baby but are on a limited budget, not to worry! Doulas who are still building up their experience or doulas in training may be just as qualified yet affordable. And most doulas, regardless of their fees, offer payment plans according to your needs.

Signs of Labor

Toward the end of your pregnancy, you may begin to experience some occasional contractions that can lead you to believe you are in labor. You may feel your belly get very hard for a few seconds, or it may feel like your baby is suddenly rolled up in a tight ball. These uterine contractions are called Braxton Hicks contractions, and they are different from those you will feel when you go into labor. Instead of "false labor," many health-care providers now refer to these as "pre-labor" contractions. Think of Braxton Hicks as practice contractions: they are not nearly strong enough to birth your baby or cause you great pain, but they can be annoying enough to keep you awake at night. Although they might become more frequent later in pregnancy, they tend to be intermittent, never developing into any pattern, and do not dilate the cervix. Some women notice them as early as 12 weeks into the pregnancy while others never feel any at all.

Since the uterus is a large muscle, you can feel it tighten and harden with Braxton Hicks as any other muscle in your body does if you contract it.

If you have numerous Braxton Hicks within a short period of time, it may be due to dehydration. Drinking a big glass of water may decrease the frequency; a change of position may do the same. If the contractions continue you should call your health-care provider, especially if you are less than 37 weeks pregnant. The signs for preterm labor are the same as the signs for full-term labor (see list on the next page). If you are experiencing any of these symptoms, contact your health-care provider for an evaluation.

BRAXTON HICKS CONTRACTIONS:

- Are usually highly irregular. For example, they can be twenty minutes apart for an hour and then all of a sudden five minutes apart, and then disappear for another hour.
- Do not get stronger or longer, or become closer together
- Usually stop when you change positions or move around
- May stop when you drink a large glass of water.

baby care tip

Timing contractions can help you determine whether or not you are actually in labor. Look at the clock and note the time from the beginning of one contraction to the beginning of the next; this is how many minutes apart your contractions are. Most health-care providers recommend that you call them when your contractions are five minutes apart.

It is important to familiarize yourself with the signs of true labor. If you're a first-time mom, you can probably expect labor to begin slowly and gradually speed up. If this is not your first child, pay close attention to the signals your body is giving you. Your labor could start and progress much more quickly because your body has done this before. The following list outlines what happens during true labor contractions.

SIGNS OF TRUE LABOR CONTRACTIONS

- Accompanied by more discomfort or pain than Braxton Hicks
- May be felt in the back
- Become progressively longer
- Become progressively stronger
- Become closer together
- Get stronger with walking
- Cause loss of mucus plug (bloody show), if it hasn't appeared already

When your contractions become longer, stronger, and closer together, there is a good chance that this is the real deal. Time your contractions for an hour or two and then call your health-care provider to report what is happening. Never hesitate to call your health-care provider at any point as you labor at home. It's far better to discuss your progression on the phone several times than to go into the hospital only to turn around and go home because you aren't far enough along (the emotional toll of which can cause labor to slow). Some other signs that your body is preparing for labor include:

- Nesting instinct (a sudden urge to clean and organize your home for the baby)
- "Lightening," or the baby "dropping" (when your belly suddenly looks lower and you may feel much more pressure on your bladder)
- Diarrhea
- Menstrual-type cramps
- Flu-like symptoms
- Lower back pain

Q. What does it mean to "lose the mucus plug"?

A. Also referred to as the bloody show, the mucus plug is mucus that forms in the cervix to close it during pregnancy. As the cervix begins to shorten (efface) and open (dilate), the plug is discharged. Sometimes small blood vessels are broken when the mucus comes loose, mixing a small amount of pink, red, or brown blood with the mucus. This bleeding is painless. The bloody show often means that labor is 24 to 72 hours away, but this is not always the case, as labor can come sooner or even weeks later. A better indicator of labor is the presence of regular contractions.

Q. My sister told me that she had the urge to clean everything in sight the day before she gave birth. At the end of my third trimester, I am the opposite—I can't even get off the couch. Is this normal?

A. Don't worry about whether or not you have the urge to "nest." Not every woman experiences this sudden burst of energy to prepare and organize the new baby's home. Some women are so exhausted during these last few weeks that the only thing they have the urge to do is lie down—and if that's how you feel, go ahead and do that!

Q. It looks like I am carrying my baby much lower this week. Has my baby moved?

A. Toward the end of your pregnancy your baby will drop, or move down into the opening of the pelvis. When your baby moves, so does the uterus, and that is why your belly looks different. For some first-time moms, this happens up to a month before the due date. For second-time moms, though, many babies don't drop until labor begins.

You may notice other changes now that your baby has dropped. For example, many pregnant women find it easier to breathe when the baby moves down, as there is less pressure on the diaphragm. You may also find that you have less heartburn. But even though your stomach may have more room, your bladder will have less, making you feel like you need to urinate more often. You may also feel more pressure in your lower back and pelvis.

Q. Is it true that I might have loose stools right before I go into labor?

A. The hormones involved in labor may contribute to loose stools a day or two before labor begins. Loose stools by themselves may or may not indicate labor. If they are accompanied by other signs of labor then call your health-care provider. But this is not a reliable symptom; you might still get loose stools from something you ate!

Q. What exactly will happen when my water breaks?

A. This is perhaps one of the most common questions asked about pregnancy and labor, probably because TV shows and movies usually depict the breaking of the water as the beginning of labor, after which chaos ensues—often a very amusing rendition of chaos. Many new parents are eager to know what this breaking feels like, when it will happen, and what they need to do when it does. Actually, most labors begin with contractions, but either way—with contractions or the release of the waters—is normal. When labor begins with the water breaking, contractions will usually start shortly thereafter. However, it could be hours before contractions begin. Conversely, your water may not break until you're approaching the end of labor.

What breaks is the amniotic sac, the bag of fluid that surrounds and cushions your baby as he or she grows. Instead of "water breaking," you may also hear the expression "rupture of the membranes," referring to the two membranes that make up the amniotic sac—the amnion and the chorion. Don't let the word "rupture" disturb you; what actually occurs is a painless tearing in the thin but strong membrane.

When they do break, the membranes will rupture either with a sudden gush or with a small, continuous trickle of fluid. It is important that you contact your health-care provider if you are leaking fluid from your vagina. Because the amniotic sac is a closed system, it is a bacteria-free place—this keeps your baby in a sterile environment. While the risk of infection is low, your health-care provider will want to monitor you and your baby more closely once there is a break in the membranes.

Q. I'm afraid that my water will break in public. If it does, will everyone around me be able to tell?

A. Relax—when your water breaks, most likely you will be the only one who notices. But every woman is different. While some will notice a gush (as if you had a bladder accident), others just notice a trickle of fluid. Since your baby's head acts somewhat like a stopper, if you do experience a gush, it is usually the fluid below the head that has come out; the rest will seep out over time. You should have time after the initial gush to change your underwear or put on a panty liner.

baby care tip

When your water breaks, note the time and the color of the fluid. Amniotic fluid should be colorless, so if it is greenish or brown in color it may contain meconium—your baby's first bowel movement. While the presence of meconium may indicate fetal distress, don't panic if you see color in the fluid. Toward the end of pregnancy, many babies pass a stool while in utero. Contact your health-care provider, who will likely have you go to the hospital right away so they can monitor you and be sure that when the baby is born, meconium doesn't go into the lungs.

Q. I am 39 weeks pregnant. When I went to my weekly prenatal visit today my doctor told me that my cervix was one centimeter dilated and 50 percent effaced and the baby was at zero station. What exactly does this mean?

A. These are terms that your health-care provider uses to describe the condition of your cervix and the vertical position of your baby in your pelvis. While an internal exam only provides a snapshot of where things are, and does not predict when you will go into labor or give birth, these measurements can be used as indicators of progress. During your vaginal exam your health-care provider felt your cervix, which is the opening of the womb, located between the vagina and the uterus (see Fig. 4-2). During labor, the cervix needs to completely thin out and open so that your baby's head can pass through into the birth canal. By checking the cervix your provider can see how much, if any, progress has been made. The process of opening is called dilation, and the process of thinning is called effacement. Dilation is measured in centimeters: When the cervix reaches ten centimeters, it is completely opened. Effacement is measured in a percentage: When the cervix is 100 percent effaced, it is completely thinned.

Your health-care provider will also check to see how low your baby is and whether he is beginning to descend into the birth canal—this is referred to as the baby's station. Stations go from minus four (when the baby has not yet entered the pelvis) to zero (when the baby's head is at the pubic bone, engaged in the pelvis) to plus four (when the baby is about to be delivered).

Q. What is the average length of a first-time labor? Some of my friends have had very short labors and some very long. Why the difference?

A. Every pregnant woman asks this question, but unfortunately it is impossible to answer. Each labor and birth is completely unique. Even different labors for the same mother can vary greatly. The average

FIGURE 4-2: Stages of cervical dilation and effacement

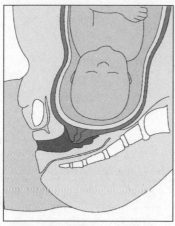

(a) Cervix before dilation or effacement

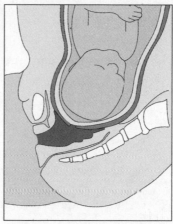

(b) Cervix is 1 to 2 cm dilated and 100% effaced

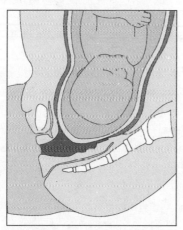

(c) Cervix is 8 to 9 cm dilated and 100% effaced with no rupture of membranes

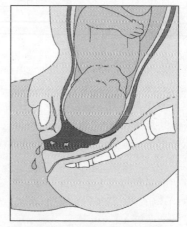

(d) Cervix is 8 to 9 cm dilated, 100% effaced, and the membranes have ruptured

length of a first-time labor is approximately twelve to fourteen hours, based on research by the American College of Obstetricians and Gynecologists (ACOG), but it is important to remember that this is just an average—some labors are longer and some are shorter. Since many factors affect the progress of labor, there is simply no way to say for sure how long yours will be. Because of the hormones involved, you will likely not be aware of the clock for the most part anyway, so it is best not to focus on the length. Labor takes however long it needs to take to birth your baby.

There are some factors that can affect the progress of labor, such as:

- The position of the baby
- A full bladder
- Fear
- Mother's position and movements during labor
- Mother's confidence and the support she receives
- Medications and medical interventions

Q. **Is there any physical preparation that I need to do before I go to the hospital, such as an enema or shaving the pubic area?**

A. No. Years ago enemas were routinely administered to women in early labor, but that practice has been dropped. The idea was that giving an enema early in labor emptied the bowels before delivery. Today the choice to receive an enema is usually up to the mother, but talk to your health-care provider during a prenatal visit if you have any questions about this. During pregnancy women often become very self-conscious and nervous about the prospect of having a bowel movement during labor. There are several reasons why you shouldn't let this thought bother you. First of all, due to the other simultaneous sensations at the time, you probably wouldn't even know if you did have one. Second, there will be disposable sheets under your bottom that can be removed very quickly and discreetly. No one but your health-care providers will see. And third, you will be so focused on birthing your baby that you likely won't give this a second thought.

In terms of shaving the pubic area, there is no medical reason to do it, so it is really up to you. If you have a cesarean birth, part of the surgical preparation will be to shave the hair where the incision will be made.

When It's Time

· · · · · · · · · · · ·

If this is your first baby, during your last weeks of pregnancy you will very likely be acutely tuned in to your body, seeking out any little sign that your baby is ready to be born. One of the most commonly asked questions I receive from expecting parents is "how will we know when it's time?" In almost all cases, you will just know. Many women feel Braxton Hicks contractions or even "real" light contractions toward the end of their pregnancies and wonder, "is this it?" As I have mentioned, if your contractions aren't regular, go away when you change positions, and do not continue for a few hours consecutively, you are probably not in labor. A lot of times, in fact, real labor contractions are a sharp contrast to those practice contractions. For many women they tend to abruptly take on a more intense feeling in the abdomen, as opposed to just a mild to moderate cramping feeling. If you do feel this change in contractions and you have any other symptoms (release of membranes, bloody show, etc.) check in with your health-care provider.

Q. I would like to stay at home as long as possible during early labor. Do you have any suggestions?

A. Especially if this is your first baby, it's a good idea to stay home as long as you feel you can. Because labor tends to progress when women feel most at ease, dilation may happen more quickly and with less chance of labor stalling if you are at home where you are comfortable. Here are a few tips to help you prepare and feel most relaxed in the midst of early labor at home.

- Talk to your partner beforehand and map out a plan for the start of your labor. Who will you call? Who will pack the bags, if they are not already packed? How will you get to the hospital when you are ready to go?
- Talk to your health-care provider beforehand about foods and drinks you can have in early labor at home. You will need as much energy as possible for labor, so it's a good idea to keep yourself hydrated and fed, particularly early on. Make sure you have those foods in the house during your last weeks of pregnancy!

- Have your favorite movie—preferably a comedy—on hand to take your mind off contractions and pass the time.

- Prior to your due date, buy a relaxation CD and get used to falling asleep and relaxing your body to it. When your contractions start getting more uncomfortable, play the CD while lying in a comfortable spot in your home. You may be able to get some sleep between contractions, which can not only help progress labor and pass time, but also give you extra energy for the upcoming marathon.

- Concentrate on relaxing to your rhythmic breathing—you will need to do this throughout labor and delivery, so it's a good idea to start right from the beginning. If you don't end up taking any childbirth classes that encourage breathing exercises, do a little research and find a few breathing techniques known to help relax women in labor (such as HypnoBirthing sleep breathing—repeatedly breathing in to the count of four and exhaling to the count of eight).

- In the weeks leading up to your due date, prepare a CD or MP3 playlist of your favorite relaxing songs. Focusing on this music can help you stay relaxed at home, in the car, and as your labor progresses.

- Remember, the key is to not panic, because fear can intensify pain. Keeping yourself as relaxed as possible will help you stay home longer and ideally progress your labor more quickly. Fear + Tension = Pain. If you can reduce your fear, the tension in your body will decrease, and therefore so will the pain.

Q. My girlfriend mentioned she had a "birth plan" when she delivered her baby. What is a birth plan, and do I need one?

A. This decision is completely up to you; it just depends on how you're feeling about your upcoming labor and birth. You do not need a birth plan. Many couples are completely satisfied with their birth experiences without ever having a "plan" in place. However, if you and your partner have strong feelings about how you would ideally like your birth to go, then it's a good idea to write them out. It's important though to think of this document as your "birth preferences" rather than a set plan. These preferences will help you communicate your wants and needs to your health-care providers but also remind you that you can never control all of the circumstances that may come up during the birth of your baby.

If you decide to make a birth plan, think about and discuss what is important to you and your partner during your labor and birth. Do you want the room lighting to be dim? Would you prefer to avoid pain medication? Are you against the idea of getting an episiotomy? Do you want to try to labor in a tub? Other items you may consider putting on your birth plan include laboring and birthing positions you are most comfortable with; the use of cameras in the room; whether you'd like a mirror to see your baby emerging; options to eat, drink, and walk during labor; fetal monitoring; use of Pitocin; use of vacuum extractor and forceps; and so on. Personalize the plan according to your own preferences; do not use a generic birth plan you came across online. Make a few copies and give one to your health-care provider during a prenatal visit so you can discuss your preferences before the birth and they can be stored in your chart. (Discussing your birth plan with your health care provider beforehand will also alert you to any hospital policies that conflict with some of your preferences.) Pack extra copies in your hospital bag so that your birth partner can share them with your care team upon arrival.

Again, it's important to keep an open mind and be flexible when it comes to your baby's birth. There will inevitably be some deviation from the plan—you may not want to walk around after all, or even think about eating! Understand that the health of you and your baby is the top priority.

baby care tip

If you hope to have an unmedicated birth and wish to have the support of your health-care providers, be sure to include that in your birth plan. This will help you focus on birthing your baby rather than the discomforts you may be experiencing during labor.

Q. My wife and I are expecting a baby any day now, and I'm worried about not making it to the hospital on time. Any advice?

A. Fathers tend to look at getting Mom to the hospital on time as their most important job, and this causes them no small amount of stress! It might make you feel better to know that the average first-time labor lasts approximately fourteen hours, so you should have plenty of time to get to the hospital when the time comes. If this is not your first baby, you will probably want to go to the hospital or at least call your health-care provider as soon as labor symptoms appear, as second-time labor can proceed rather quickly.

Get yourself organized by making a list of things that you will need when you leave for the hospital (or even pack these things early) including insurance cards, fully charged camera and/or batteries, a list of phone numbers of people you will call after the baby is born, toiletries, and clothes for each member of the family. That way, when your partner is in labor and far enough along, the only thing you'll need to do is drive.

A few weeks before the due date, it's a good idea to drive to the hospital and become familiar with the route, parking, and entrance areas. Many hospitals offer valet parking for a nominal fee—check this out beforehand. Keep your gas tank full, and think about alternate routes in case of a traffic tie-up. Don't speed—getting into a fender-bender will only slow you down!

baby care tip

In the midst of labor and birth you may find yourself in a scenario you had not envisioned—e.g., your labor isn't progressing, your baby has turned breech, or your baby's heartbeat has slowed. Just remember that, aside from very rare emergencies, in most cases there will be time to rationally discuss your options. If you and your partner would like to be actively involved in these discussions and given time alone to consider the next step, indicate that on your birth plan. Some parents I work with would rather leave any medical decisions completely up to their health-care providers, while others prefer to be an active part of all decisions. While either is perfectly fine, it never hurts to be aware of the various options.

As you prepare for the arrival of your baby, whether it is quelling aches of late pregnancy, practicing relaxation techniques for early labor, or discussing strategy with your partner, remember that this is an amazing juncture in your life. Seek out positive messages about pregnancy, labor, and birth, and tune out the negative! This will help you to relax before, during, and after the birth of your baby and will allow you to enjoy every stage more fully. Just trust your body and the inner wisdom that occurs during the birth process. In addition be sure to communicate with your birth partner and health-care providers—they will all be there to help guide you through once you arrive at your hospital to meet your baby.

· 5 ·

Labor and Birth

If you're like many parents I've helped through labor, you will feel a sense of relief upon arriving at the hospital in labor. Your health-care providers will be there to guide you through the labor and birthing process as well as help to ensure the safety of you and your baby. However, familiarizing yourselves beforehand with labor-easing techniques and birth-associated medical procedures and terminology will help make your overall hospital birthing experience a positive one. What you learn in a childbirth class will prepare you for birth itself, but not necessarily for the hospital experience. I've been so fortunate to be a part of hundreds of births alongside laboring women and their partners. Each one has been unique but they all share a common thread—their desire to have a healthy baby and an enjoyable birthing and postpartum experience. In this chapter I will address common questions first-time parents have about what to expect at the hospital, as well as share tips on how to manage a comfortable labor and delivery of your baby.

Checking In

Expert advice on pregnancy and birth very rarely focuses on the logistics of what happens when you get to the hospital and what you can expect as labor progresses. But these seemingly minor details matter—your baby is about to be born! Here's a heads-up on what you might generally expect upon admitting and thereafter.

Q. Will my wife be admitted into a labor room as soon as we arrive at the hospital?

A. Probably not, unless she is about to deliver, which is highly unusual. After you park your car you will most likely go to the Obstetrical/Maternity registration desk. If you've taken a tour of the hospital, you should know how to find it; if not, ask at the main hospital desk for directions to OB admitting. Most hospitals have staff available to point you in the right direction. It's a good idea to preregister so that you can avoid dealing with a lot of paperwork when you arrive in labor; you may receive a registration packet from your health-care provider during your second trimester, and sometimes their office will process the registration for you. Sending this information to the hospital ahead of time expedites the process, but don't worry if you forgot or couldn't preregister—just make sure to bring your insurance card so the hospital administrator can get the information into the billing system. If in doubt, call the hospital and your insurance carrier a few weeks beforehand to find out if there will be a copay upon admission and how much it will be.

The admitting process doesn't take long, and often your partner can take care of it. When you're finished, someone from admitting will either walk you to the labor and delivery floor or show you how to get there. And don't worry if you miss the admitting department altogether. The unit secretary will usually be able to supply them with the information they need. They'll understand you have other things on your mind during this time!

baby care tip

Learn about the hospital's parking arrangements before you arrive in labor. Some hospitals have garages, while others have valet parking, and some have both. Find out where you should park and what the costs are.

Q. My health-care provider told me to go to the triage area on the labor floor when I come in. What is a triage area?

A. Triage is an area on the labor and delivery floor where your health-care provider determines whether or not you are far enough along in labor to be admitted into the hospital. Your cervix will be checked for dilation and effacement and your contractions will be monitored. If it is determined that you are in labor, you will be admitted to a labor and delivery room. If you are not in labor, a care plan will be developed based upon your needs. You may be sent home with some suggestions on how to stimulate your labor.

---

baby care tip

Bring a book or magazine with you to the hospital. Sometimes the triage area is very busy, and unless you are in active labor you may be waiting for several hours before your providers come up with a plan of care for you. It's best to have something positive on which to focus your energy!

Q. What can I expect the hospital room to look like?

A. There are two basic types of maternity rooms—LDR (labor, delivery, and recovery) and LDRP (labor, delivery, recovery, and postpartum). Check with your hospital to find out which types of rooms they offer. Many larger birthing hospitals tend to have LDR rooms, in which you will labor, deliver, and spend a few hours recovering before being transferred to a postpartum room, where you will remain for the rest of your hospital stay. A labor and delivery nurse will support you for the birth and a postpartum nurse will monitor you and your baby after you are transferred. If you birth in an LDRP room, you will remain in the same room for your entire hospital stay.

Both options will generally be very comfortable for you, your partner, and your baby. Labor rooms have birthing beds that adjust for use in a variety of positions during labor and delivery. These rooms are typically decorated in a way that feels homey, but with all the necessary technology to ensure a safe delivery should any complication arise. All methods of pain relief, including epidurals, are available in both types of rooms. Many rooms have rocking chairs, a bed for the partner, a refrigerator, and closets and drawers for your belongings. Your hospital room will have a bathroom with a shower and perhaps even a tub. If you haven't taken a tour, you will probably be surprised at how warm and cozy your labor room looks. Everything you need to birth your baby will be in this room, and it will probably look even cozier after you've given birth.

baby care tip

Do yourself a favor and don't bring unnecessary things to the hospital. Most rooms, whether LDR or LDRP, are small and get quite crowded. Limit yourself to the basics recommended in chapter 1. One or two bags are all that is necessary. It may be easier to fit everything in one bag; if not, you can pack a labor bag and a postpartum bag. You do not need your baby's car seat or postpartum bag when you arrive. After the baby is born, your partner can take some things home and bring you back some postpartum supplies if needed. The less you bring to the hospital, the easier it will be when you're getting ready to leave. As new parents, you'll have enough to think about when you take your baby home without having to worry about several suitcases!

First Stage of Labor

Labor has four different stages. During the first stage, contractions ripen (that is, open) your cervix in preparation for birth until it is ten centimeters dilated. This stage is further divided into three phases—early, active, and transition. For most women the early phase, when the cervix is between one to three centimeters in dilation, is the longest stage, and then things tend to pick up around five centimeters' dilation. Transition marks the end of stage one and the beginning of stage two. Once your cervix is fully dilated and effaced, the second stage consists of pushing and ends with the birth of your baby. The third stage is the birth of the placenta: within about a half hour of your baby being born, the placenta will detach from the wall of your uterus and be "born."

There is also a fourth stage of labor, which lasts for a few hours after birth or until you and your baby are stable. The fourth stage is the period from the time the placenta is delivered until the uterus remains firm on its own. During this time, the uterus will stabilize and begin to return to its nonpregnant state. Your nurse will check your uterus frequently to make sure it is starting to contract.

Let's take a look at the three stages in more detail. Once you understand the stages of labor, you'll have a better sense of what actions will be most helpful during each stage.

EARLY LABOR:

AT HOME

Cervical dilation: one to three centimeters

▶ **WHAT MOM CAN DO**

- Move around
- Walk
- Change positions frequently
- Favor upright positions
- Eat lightly
- Hydrate, hydrate, hydrate

▶ **WHAT PARTNER CAN DO**

- Time contractions
- Make sure bag is packed
- Help Mom to relax
- Introduce pleasurable distractions
- Call health-care provider, but be prepared to let Mom speak directly

EARLY LABOR STORY

In order to get a sense of the different ways a labor can start and progress, it can be valuable to hear firsthand labor experiences from other moms. I spent time over a year speaking with hundreds of new moms, asking them to share some of their memories from labor. Here are the early labor accounts two moms shared with me.

"Contractions started at 5 AM and were about twelve minutes apart. They were strong, but I was still able to take a quick shower and have a light breakfast after I called my doctor. By 9 AM the contractions were about five minutes apart, so we packed the car and drove to the hospital. By then the contractions were very intense and I could barely walk. We stopped by OB admitting and then walked to the labor floor. I thought I would be embarrassed about all the moaning and groaning I was doing, but I really did not care about anything but the contractions. We arrived on the labor floor and when they checked me, I was already four centimeters dilated."

—Angela, age twenty-eight

"My contractions started at 10 PM but were about eight to fifteen minutes apart and very irregular. I called my midwife and was told to try to get some rest but to call if the contractions became closer together. I dozed on and off but could not really sleep at all. At 6 AM I called my midwife again because I was still having contractions but they were not getting more intense. She told me to come to the hospital for an evaluation. Upon arriving at the hospital I was sent to the triage area. A nurse checked my cervix and told me I was almost two centimeters dilated and 50 percent effaced. By this time the contractions had slowed down quite a bit—about every fifteen minutes, and they were not as strong. I was told I could either go back home and wait for labor to progress or I could walk around the hospital to see if that would help move things along. At 9 AM I decided to go back home since we lived less than twenty minutes away. I had almost no sleep the night before, so once I was back in my bed I fell asleep for two hours. I woke up and immediately felt a contraction. This felt much more intense than the earlier contractions. At eleven thirty we went back to the hospital and when the nurse checked my cervix again I was happy to hear that I was almost five centimeters."

—Keri, age thirty-two

ACTIVE LABOR

Cervical dilation: four to eight centimeters

▶ **WHAT MOM CAN DO**

- Go to hospital
- Begin breathing techniques
- Practice relaxation techniques
- Use birthing ball
- Sit in rocking chair
- Walk
- Change positions frequently
- Take warm shower or bath
- Sip water or fluids

▶ **WHAT PARTNER CAN DO**

- Support Mom physically and emotionally
- Give massages
- Eliminate distractions (e.g., cell phones and TV)
- Give Mom praise and encouragement

ACTIVE LABOR STORIES

When I speak with first-time moms about their active labor experiences, most instantly recall the way they best eased the increasingly intense contractions, whether it was using the shower or a birthing ball or practicing breathing and relaxation techniques they learned in a birthing class. Here's what three of those moms recalled about active labor.

"The contractions got really strong as labor progressed. Moving around and changing positions helped me to get through them. My favorite place to be was sitting on a birthing ball in the shower."
—Amanda, age twenty-six

"I remember that I didn't feel like talking to anyone anymore. In early labor I was chatting with the nurses and joking with my partner but all of a sudden I felt like concentrating on the contractions and just birthing my baby." **—Theresa, age thirty-four**

"The contractions started to get very intense, and what really helped me get through them was my husband coaching me to breathe. I felt like holding my breath for some reason, but he reminded me how important it was to breathe slowly through each contraction. So I did!" **—Hope, age twenty-seven**

Many hospitals have birthing balls available for your use, so before you bring your own, ask if you can use one where you're giving birth. Have your nurse bring one to the room for you, and then just sit and rock back and forth. Alternate between rocking in a chair and moving on the birthing ball. Walk (even if just around the nurses' station); get into squats and hands and knees positions, slow dance—whatever feels good. Ask your nurse or health-care provider if you can use the shower or a tub. If your hospital does not have a tub, use a shower chair and let the hot water massage your back. If you prefer to be discreet in the water, bring something comfortable to wear from home, wrap a towel around you, or just use a hospital gown.

TRANSITION

Cervical dilation: eight to ten centimeters

▶ **WHAT MOM CAN DO**

- Take one contraction at a time
- Rest between contractions
- Ice chips between contractions
- Remember transition goes quickly

▶ **WHAT PARTNER CAN DO**

- Provide encouragement
- Help Mom to focus
- Help Mom to get into a comfortable position
- Remind her this is the shortest phase

TRANSITION STORIES

Like every stage of labor, the transition stage is different for every woman. Some get through it quickly and relatively easily depending on the techniques or medications used, while it can be more challenging for others. The common thread though, in speaking with so many new moms over the past year, was that the transition stage was a powerful experience. No matter what they felt physically during that stage, most expressed the overwhelming feeling they had knowing they were soon going to meet their babies. Here are a few of those stories about the transition stage:

> "This was definitely the hardest part of labor, but it was also the shortest. I went from eight to ten centimeters in about an hour, thankfully."
>
> **—Eldi, age thirty**

> "My body started shaking when I neared ten centimeters, and my nurse told me that was normal. Clenching my teeth together and saying the alphabet slowly helped me to deal with the shaking."
>
> **—Tara, age twenty-nine**

> "I'm not sure why, but all of a sudden I started yelling at my husband. He was so loving and helpful throughout the pregnancy and the labor, but right then, all I wanted to think about was how I was going to get through the next contraction. What really helped is when my husband let me squeeze his hand during each contraction."
>
> **—Leah, age twenty-five**

baby care tip

Having the freedom to move around can help you deal with the discomforts of labor, and further assist your pelvis in widening to help move baby through the birth canal.

If you are not connected to the fetal monitor during your labor, go ahead and walk the halls of the hospital. If your hospital has stairs, walk up and down them. These movements will help to put pressure on your cervix, which will help your labor to progress.

Make sure to let your labor nurse know that you're interested in walking—this is something you can add to your birth plan. Your nurse or health-care provider will monitor your baby's heart rate according to hospital protocol, possibly every hour or every half hour. This is sometimes done with a device called a Doppler, a handheld ultrasound device that detects the baby's heartbeat (see tip on page 126).

If your baby needs continuous fetal monitoring, ask your nurse or caregiver if you can use a telemetry unit. Telemetry is a form of wireless fetal monitoring that allows you to be continuously monitored without being connected to a machine. The benefit is that you have full freedom to move around without the constricting wires. Not all hospitals have this equipment, though, so you may want to find out ahead of time.

Coping with Contractions

Birthing ball—In addition to relieving discomfort during pregnancy, the birthing ball is also a highly recommended tool for laboring moms. The swaying motion when sitting on the ball opens the pelvic joints, which helps the baby rotate and descend.

Rocking chair—Sitting in a rocking chair tends to be a soothing motion for moms. Try inhaling and exhaling slowly along with the rocking motion, which can help keep you focused on breathing steadily through tough contractions. As with the birthing ball, sitting allows gravity to put pressure on your pelvis and cervix, helping your body further prepare for the birth of your baby.

Slow dancing—Swaying back and forth can help change the shape of the pelvis, allow gravity to slowly move your baby downward, and alleviate some of the pressure you feel during labor. Slow dancing with your partner also creates intimacy in the moment, which can help relax you.

FIGURE 5-1(a–f): Women in six labor positions

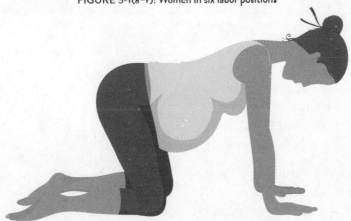

(a) hands and knees

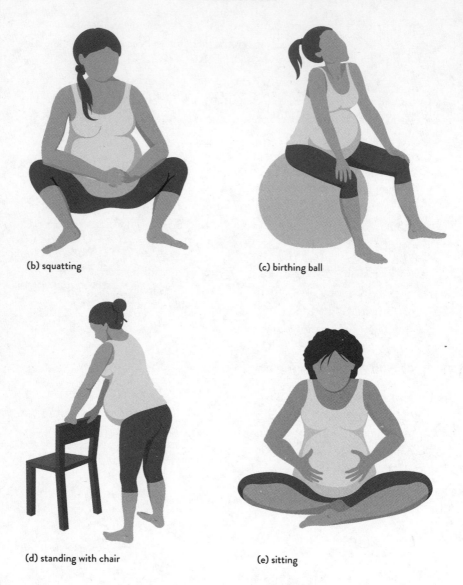

(b) squatting

(c) birthing ball

(d) standing with chair

(e) sitting

Shower or tub—Ask your health-care provider if you can sit on a chair or a birthing ball in the shower. The warm spray of the shower on your back or belly can be very comforting.

Squatting and lunging—These positions open the pelvic joints and create space for the baby to descend. A prenatal yoga class may help increase your strength and flexibility during pregnancy, making these positions easier during labor.

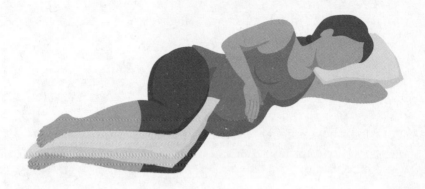

(f) side lying

Abdominal breathing—Breathe in through your nose or mouth and exhale through your mouth. Fill your lungs completely during inhalation and then exhale completely for the most efficient oxygenation for you and your baby.

Massage—Moderate to deep massage can help relieve leg cramps and other muscle tension during labor.

Light touch—When the birth partner lightly touches the skin it causes a release of endorphins, which decrease your pain sensation. Lightly touch the abdominal skin directly over the uterus for the same benefits.

Aromatherapy—Lavender and rosemary oils are especially relaxing. Some women find that the scent of lemon or peppermint can reduce nausea.

Music—Soft, rhythmic music or sounds of nature can help you "stay in the zone" and relax.

Hydrotherapy—Water from the shower or in a tub can be very relaxing and works well, especially when labor is active.

Second Stage of Labor: Birth

. . . .

The second stage of labor, also known as the pushing stage, begins when your cervix is fully dilated and completely effaced, and your baby has descended into the birth canal. Your contractions during this stage will feel different than the contractions you felt during stage one. When a contraction begins, you may or may not have an immediate urge to bear down, but it will bring you relief to push. Between contractions, you should be relatively comfortable; in fact, your body releases endorphins during this time that will calm and relax you between contractions.

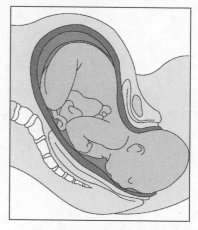

FIGURE 5-2: Baby's head crowning

Your baby's position within your pelvis will determine when the urge to push begins. Moving into a more upright position usually brings on the urge to push more quickly. The urge to bear down and push will become stronger as your baby moves further into the vagina. If you have back labor—in which the pain of contractions is felt in the lower back—experiment with different positions such as side lying, hands and knees, and standing. Believe it or not, many women also get a burst of energy as the birth of the baby nears!

Your health-care providers will direct you to respond to the urge to bear down, but it's also important to follow your body's lead and push for as long as you feel the urge. Your partner and health-care provider will be coaching and encouraging you during most of this stage. Once the contraction is over, you should breathe lightly and rest until the next one comes.

If you have had anesthesia, spontaneous pushing may not be possible because you cannot feel the contractions. Your birth partner, nurse, or health-care provider will tell you when and for how long to push. Don't worry; you will get the hang of it very quickly.

Birth is near when your baby's head crowns, meaning that the top of the head has emerged so far that it no longer retreats between pushes. You will most likely feel a stinging or burning sensation as the muscle stretches around the baby's head, but it doesn't last very long. Your birth attendant will direct your pushes and support your perineum until your baby's head emerges, and then your baby will gradually rotate to the side (this helps the shoulders to slip through the pelvis). After one shoulder emerges, the rest of your baby's body will deliver rather quickly. Your baby will most likely be placed on your chest while the rest of the delivery is completed. Soon after the birth, the umbilical cord will be clamped in two places and then cut by either your health-care provider or partner.

Q. As an expectant father/partner I always thought I would want to cut my baby's umbilical cord, but now I'm not so sure. Do other new parents feel this way?

A. Yes, you can rest assured that you are not alone. Whether or not to cut the umbilical cord is a personal decision and varies greatly from family to family For some fathers/partners, cutting the cord makes them feel involved in their baby's birth and can be a very powerful experience. For others, cutting the cord is not something that they are particularly interested in or comfortable with. Whatever you choose, try not to put pressure on yourself. Do what you feel is right for you.

Q. Many of our friends have banked cord blood. Is this routinely recommended?

A. Because the science behind stem cell treatments is still emerging, cord blood banking is not routinely recommended, unless there is a family medical need for a stem cell transplantation or a family is looking to donate for philanthropic reasons. That said, it is a personal decision and there are several options, should you chose to do so.

Cord blood is the remaining blood found in a baby's umbilical cord and the placenta at birth. Because it's rich in hematopoietic stem cells—which can produce new blood cells for potentially life-saving treatments at a later date—some parents decide to collect and store it in a private or public cord blood bank.

Public cord blood banks are free to donate to, are run by nonprofit organizations, and can be found throughout the United States. When a family adds their baby's cord blood into a public bank, it is not stored for their personal use, but it may, after testing, come to help another person if shown to be a good match in fighting a particular disease. If the donating baby grows up to need cord blood for a treatment, they have the possibility of receiving a donation from the public bank.

Private cord blood banks cost money, but with this method the cord blood is stored and reserved for the donating family's use. It is important to note, however, that should a need for a cord blood treatment arise, it is not always guaranteed that one's own cord blood, or that of a sibling, will be beneficial. The type of blood needed depends on what kind of disease requires treating. In fact, according to the American College of Obstetricians and Gynecologists (ACOG) Committee Opinion in 2015, "Most conditions potentially treated by a patient's own umbilical cord blood already exist in his or her own cells and, therefore, the stored blood cannot be used to treat the same individual."[12] If the family's stored cord blood will not provide effective treatment, private cord blood banks arrange for alternative donations provided a match is found. Before you sign on with a private cord blood bank, make sure to do your research and understand all of the fees and steps involved.

It may seem like the decisions you have to make about your baby's birth are endless, and by now you have probably been overwhelmed with cord blood banking brochures, magazine ads, and online stories that tap into your emotions. But try not to let these marketing messages pressure you or make you feel guilty, whatever you decide. Simply sit down with your health-care provider or your baby's pediatrician, ask questions, and weigh their answers and recommendations carefully. Here are few to get you started:

- What diseases could my baby's own cord blood help treat for themselves or their siblings down the line?
- In what circumstances might my baby's cord blood not be helpful in treating disease?

12   American College of Obstetricians and Gynecologists, "Umbilical Cord Blood Banking," Committee Opinion no. 648 (December 2015). acog.org.

- Are you affiliated with any for-profit umbilical cord blood banking companies that may present a conflict of interest in your advice on this matter?
- Are there any circumstances during birth that might prevent the collection of cord blood?
- What happens to my baby's cord blood once it's collected?

baby care tip

Partners—whether or not to cut the umbilical cord is a personal decision. Think about whether you want to do this and let the health-care provider know. Do not feel pressured. You might be surprised to learn that many partners decide to leave the cutting to the medical staff.

SECOND STAGE LABOR STORIES

Many of the first-time moms I have cared for confess that when they got pregnant, the second or "pushing stage" of labor seemed like the most intimidating part of labor for them. Because they'd seen so many images of women in agonizing pain pushing their babies out in TV and film, they just took those images as representative of the "real thing." That's why it can be helpful to hear moms verbalize the experience themselves, as three of the women I spoke with have below:

"It took me a while to get used to pushing. I didn't feel comfortable holding my legs up and apart, but I got used to it pretty quickly. I pushed for about an hour and a half and then my provider told me my baby was crowning. Two more pushes and there she was—our beautiful baby girl." **—Caroline, age thirty**

"I was afraid to push at first, but then when I did I noticed it felt better to push than not to. I pushed better with my eyes closed. After almost three hours of pushing, the final few moments had finally arrived. I felt a lot of pressure as his head was being born but only for a few seconds. I was so happy when our son was born." **—Laurette, age twenty-six**

"I didn't think I would be able to push my baby out because I couldn't feel the contractions at all. My nurse told me when to push, how hard to push, and for how long. It took me two or three contractions before I got the hang of it. It was hard work for about two hours but I got the best reward of all when it was all over—my baby."

—Karen, age twenty-nine

baby care tip

As you're pushing, try to keep your mouth open—don't hold your breath. This will help you to push more effectively. When your contraction is over, take a big, cleansing breath and let yourself relax.

Third and Fourth Stages of Labor

The third stage of labor refers to the period following the delivery of your baby. This is the shortest and least painful stage, lasting about ten to thirty minutes. The pain of labor goes away but you may feel some uterine contractions as the placenta separates. You may also feel an urge to bear down and push the placenta out. Once the placenta is delivered, the uterus will contract and close off the open blood vessels. Your health-care provider may administer oxytocin after delivery to encourage the uterus to contract firmly. Many women don't even notice when the placenta has been delivered, and for others it's just a quick feeling of pressure. Your health-care provider may ask if you'd like to see it, and if you want to, go ahead. It's been supporting your baby inside you for nine months!

The fourth stage of labor begins after the umbilical cord is cut and lasts until your condition is stable and your uterus is firm, usually an hour or two. Your health-care providers will monitor your blood pressure, pulse, respirations, temperature, lochia (vaginal discharge), and uterine tone. Your perineum will be checked for swelling and bleeding. You will probably be feeling euphoric with your new baby. Some women cannot wait to hold their babies, while other women need a few minutes or more to process the birth and get used to not being in labor anymore. It usually does not take long for your baby to become the center of your world!

baby care tip

Breastfeeding is a great way to help your uterus to contract after birth. Another way to encourage uterine contraction is to massage the top part of the uterus, called the fundus. It should feel firm, not soft. If the uterus does not feel firm, there may be a clot inside. Your health-care provider will apply continued gentle pressure on the uterus following massage until it begins to feel firm.

Pain Medication in Labor

Whether or not to use pain relief medications in labor is completely up to you. Every woman copes with labor in a unique way. Some women choose to have an unmedicated childbirth and others decide ahead of time that they would like to use medications. Circumstances may occur during labor—including the baby's position, the degree of dilation and effacement, and the intensity and length of your labor—that will influence your decision, as well as your hospital's options for pain management. Every woman's perception of pain varies and every labor is unique, just as every baby is unique. One first-time mom in my childbirth class asked me how she could make sure she could get an epidural right away upon hospital admission. She was so worried about the potential pain and thought she would not be able to bear any part of the childbirth. We discussed what her body is capable of and what she can do to help decrease pain (techniques I will discuss a bit later). As it turned out she came into the hospital when she was already seven centimeters. Labor progressed quickly—after getting out of the shower at the hospital she was almost fully dilated. Her twins were born soon after and she used no medications! In this case, she was initially adamant about getting an epidural but when she was actually in labor she realized it was not necessary. If you find that the opposite is true for you there are several options for pain medication.

The type of pain medication you can receive depends on where you are in the labor process. Pain medication in early labor will affect a woman very differently than pain medication later on, just as a medication recommended in early labor may not be recommended during the pushing stage. This chart and the questions that follow will address what pain medications work best during each stage of labor. Try to learn about pain medications before you are in labor so you know all your options and can make the choices that feel right for you.

Pain medications used in labor have specific characteristics that make them appropriate at certain times. There are typically two types of medication—systemic and regional anesthetics. Systemic medications can be taken orally or can be injected into a muscle so that they go into your bloodstream. Because they are absorbed into your bloodstream, they affect your entire body. These medications do cross over to your baby through the placenta, but most babies experience no or very few side effects (see pages 118–20).

Regional anesthetics are used to numb a specific area of the body—particularly the legs, stomach, and lower chest for labor, vaginal birth, and C-sections. Types of regional anesthetics include epidurals, spinals, and combined spinal-epidurals, all of which are injected into the spinal canal to relieve any painful sensations. A spinal injection has a more immediate effect than an epidural because it is injected directly into the spine's fluid sac, as opposed to an epidural, which is injected into the area around the fluid sac.[13]

MEDICATIONS IN LABOR

Stage One

▶ **SLEEPING AID** (Seconal, Ambien)

- **HOW IT'S GIVEN:** Usually by mouth, but occasionally IM (into muscle) or IV (into vein)
- **DURATION OF EFFECT:** four to six hours
- **EFFECTS ON MOM:** Promotes relaxation so you can rest and sleep very early in labor. Will make you tired and drowsy, but can also make you nauseous.
- **EFFECTS ON BABY:** Very little if given early in labor, but if given late in labor baby may be "sleepy," with possible respiratory depression.

---

13 J. M. Carabuena and B. S. Kodali, "Anesthesia for Cesarean Delivery," Pain Relief Options During Childbirth, painfreebirthing.com/english/cs.htm.

▶ **NARCOTIC** (Nubain or similar medication such as Stadol, Fentanyl, Demerol, or morphine, depending on the preferences of your hospital)

- **HOW IT'S GIVEN:** Either IM or IV
- **DURATION OF EFFECT:** three to six hours
- **EFFECTS ON MOM:** Helps take the edge off; provides some relief during peaks of contractions; may relax you and make you sleepy. Occasionally may cause nausea, vomiting, or feeling of being disoriented. Some women may experience hypotension, a drop in blood pressure.
- **EFFECTS ON BABY:** Very few effects on baby if given four hours or more before birth. However, some babies may experience respiratory depression (difficulty breathing) and may appear very sleepy if medication administered one to three hours before birth.

▶ **EPIDURAL**

- **HOW IT'S GIVEN:** Given in active labor while you are lying on your side or sitting. Lower back is cleaned with antiseptic wash, and a small local anesthetic is given to numb the area. Once the area is numbed, a regional anesthetic is introduced. Needle is introduced though the numbed area of skin into epidural space and a thin flexible plastic catheter inserted. Catheter is left in place for continuous administration or in case additional medication is needed. Takes about five to ten minutes to administer.
- **DURATION OF EFFECT:** Because the catheter remains in place and anesthetic medication is infused continuously, the pain relief will last throughout labor. Many hospitals now use "patient-controlled epidural anesthesia," which allows you to control with a switch how much pain medication you receive.
- **EFFECTS ON MOM:** The pain from contractions will be mostly or completely relieved because the area will be numb. You will be completely awake and alert during labor. In order to prevent a drop in blood pressure, you will be given IV fluids. Since you may not feel the urge to urinate, you will most likely have a urinary catheter to keep your bladder empty.
- **EFFECTS ON BABY:** Research inconclusive. There are no known side effects.

▶ **NITROUS OXIDE (N_2O):**

- **HOW IT'S GIVEN:** N_2O is self-administered and has a rapid onset of about thirty seconds, which correlates with volume and rate of inhalation. N_2O administration is intermittent and delivered via face mask.

- **DURATION OF EFFECT:** As soon as the mask is taken off and you take a few deep breaths, the gas is cleared from your body.
- **EFFECTS ON MOM:** Side effects may include sedation, dizziness, nausea, and vomiting.
- **EFFECTS ON BABY:** Research inconclusive. There are no known side effects.

▶ **INTRATHECAL (SPINAL CANAL) NARCOTIC**

- **HOW IT'S GIVEN:** During active labor, a narcotic is injected into the subarachnoid space, which contains spinal fluid
- **DURATION OF EFFECT:** Takes effect almost immediately and lasts up to two hours
- **EFFECTS ON MOM:** Rapid onset of pain relief. You will be completely awake and alert. May not last through second stage of labor, but addition of epidural catheter allows more medication to be given, so pain relief can last throughout labor.
- **EFFECTS ON BABY:** See epidural effects, above.

Stage Two (if epidural not already administered)

▶ **LOCAL ANESTHETIC** (most commonly lidocaine)

- **HOW IT'S GIVEN:** Injection into the perineum prior to an episiotomy
- **DURATION OF EFFECT:** Lasts approximately twenty to thirty minutes
- **EFFECTS ON MOM:** Numbs vagina and perineum for episiotomy or when forceps and vacuum are used for delivery
- **EFFECTS ON BABY:** None.

Q. What if I try all of the nonpharmacological methods for pain relief and then decide I would like an epidural? Will this slow my labor down?

A. An epidural is anesthesia, which causes some numbness of the legs. Most modern-day epidurals (compared to those used years ago) result in very little motor block, so most women can fully move their legs, move around in bed, and push during labor, but may just be a bit weak and not safely able to walk. You may hear the term "walking epidural," but very few women with epidurals actually walk.

It is because of this limited mobility that labor can slow down after the epidural is administered. Walking, movement, and laboring in different positions all help labor to progress. Also, women with an epidural may not feel the instinctual urge to push, which may make for a less effective second stage of labor.

However, most recent research shows that labor is only minimally slowed with the use of modern-day epidural anesthesia. If labor does slow, it can be hard to pinpoint the epidural medication as the sole cause, as many factors combine to determine how fast or slow a particular labor progresses. Recent surveys show that 50 to 75 percent of U.S. women receive epidural anesthesia in childbirth. Of course, any medication carries risks, so be sure to weigh those with the benefits and ask your health-care provider and the anesthesiologist any questions you may have.

Q. My doctor recommended that I use an analgesic or narcotic before I get my epidural. What is that and what will it do?

A. Unlike the epidural, narcotics do not take the pain away but rather are known to "take the edge off." Your health-care provider may suggest using these first because they might provide enough relief and are less restricting than the epidural. Or she may recommend the narcotic if you are still in very early labor, and she would prefer your labor be more active before administering an epidural. There are some advantages to the narcotic—even though you will have an IV (see page 125) and continuous monitoring, the narcotic does not require you to stay in bed. You may be somewhat limited in your movement due to the cords, but you often can still sit on the birthing ball or rocking chair, or even get into some hands-and-knees or squatting positions. All medications have risks for mom and baby, so be sure to thoroughly discuss your options before making choices.

Medical Interventions in Childbirth

No one can predict what your labor and delivery will be like. All we know, as I've said, is that every labor and birth experience is unique. Your labor will be different from the labor your mother or your sister had, and each of your own labor experiences will be different. Most labors go smoothly and many go as planned, but occasionally medical interventions may be necessary to ensure a safe delivery. An intervention in labor is something your health-care provider may recommend in order to identify, prevent, or treat a medical concern, and it is important to familiarize yourself with some of the most common choices. Talk to your health-care provider ahead of time about interventions that are routinely used and about any concerns you may have. The following section gives you an overview of the interventions you may face during your labor and delivery including induction of labor, intravenous fluids (IV), fetal monitoring, amniotomy (breaking of the waters), and delivery by forceps and vacuum extractor.

Induction and Augmentation of Labor

Your labor may be induced for a medical reason, such as preeclampsia or diabetes, or if continuing the pregnancy is a risk to either you or your baby. There are also fetal conditions that may make induction necessary, such as a baby who isn't growing enough in the uterus, a placenta that is not functioning effectively, or a situation in which your amniotic sac has ruptured but you don't start contractions within twenty-four hours. You might also have your labor induced if your due date comes and goes and there is no sign that your cervix and baby are ready for birth. Situations like these may make it necessary to help your body begin the process of labor, although some are more open to discussion with health-care providers, while others are medically necessary. According to American College of Obstetricians and Gynecologists, about 20 percent of labors in the United States are induced.

Labor is generally induced through intravenous medication called Pitocin. Based on the condition of your cervix, your health-care provider may begin the Pitocin drip right away or may decide to apply a prostaglandin gel or suppository to help soften your cervix in preparation for the Pitocin. Induction is usually more successful on a cervix that has been softened.

While Pitocin is administered through an IV, it doesn't necessarily restrict you to a bed. It does tend to create contractions that are closer together and stronger than they would be naturally, and this can make for a more challenging labor for both you and your baby. Because of this, you will have continuous fetal monitoring with Pitocin—just to keep an eye on how your baby is handling the labor.

If your health-care provider mentions or suggests an induction, take the time to discuss the reasons as well as the risks involved. Some risks your health-care provider will discuss with you include a failed induction, increased risk of a cesarean section (especially if this is the mother's first birth and she has an unripe cervix), increased risk of fetal distress, and hyperstimulation of the uterus.

Q. It is almost two weeks past my due date and my health-care provider is talking about inducing my labor with Pitocin. Why might induction be necessary, and what is this medication?

A. Pitocin is the synthetic form of oxytocin, a hormone your body produces to stimulate uterine contractions. Pitocin is administered with an IV (intravenous infusion) pump so its dosage can be carefully controlled. The Pitocin will stimulate your uterus to contract and ideally cause your cervix to dilate. During the induction your labor will be continuously monitored, and you will have close nursing care to ensure safe administration. This is important because there are some risks, such as uterine hyperstimulation and fetal distress. Discuss the risks and disadvantages of this medication, along with any other concerns you might have, with your health-care provider prior to labor.

Your health-care provider may recommend induction for the following cases:

- You are one to two weeks past your estimated due date. The placenta may become less effective at this point and may stop providing necessary nutrients to your baby, which may increase your risk for a cesarean birth.
- Your water breaks and your labor doesn't start on its own, putting you and your baby at risk for developing an infection
- Your baby is not thriving and growing as he should, or you have too little amniotic fluid.
- You develop preeclampsia or a chronic illness that may threaten your or your baby's health.

Q. My labor is progressing well, but all of a sudden my contractions slow down. My health-care provider recommends that we augment my labor with Pitocin. Why did my labor stall, and what is augmentation?

A. There are many reasons why your labor could have stalled. It could be your baby's position, tension or fear in your mind and body, or just part of the natural ebb and flow of your labor. Things will likely pick up on their own if given time and patience, provided the baby is doing well. Your nurse can recommend nonpharmacological ways to encourage your labor to get going again. However, if it is determined that it would be best to move things along, Pitocin is commonly used for this purpose.

baby care tip

If this is your first baby you may be looking for ways to help move labor along. Here are some techniques that may help you to stimulate your labor, many of which may also help you cope with contractions.

- Change positions. Your movement will help your baby get into a different position, which may be all that is needed to speed things up. For example, if you've been in bed or rocking in a chair for thirty minutes, get up and start walking.
- Stand up, sway, and rock. These movements help labor to progress by the effects of gravity. When you stand up, your baby's head is able to apply more pressure to the cervix, which can help dilation and effacement.
- Sit on a birthing ball and move your hips and buttocks in a figure-eight motion.

Remember that as long as you and baby are doing well, there might not be a reason to "move things along" just yet. Sometimes labor is meant to take a little longer. Try to relax.

Amniotomy

Q. I am in labor, my contractions are slowing down, and my health-care provider is talking about breaking my water. Will this speed up my labor? Will this procedure hurt?

A. It may or may not speed up your labor. Amniotomy, or artificial rupture of the membranes, is generally not painful. In a relatively quick procedure, the amniotic sac is punctured with a plastic tool that is inserted through the opening in the cervix and then quickly removed. It is a common misconception that the waters always break at the beginning of labor. In fact, they can release at any time—often near the end of labor, in fact, when the baby's head tends to be low. Your waters will release on their own at some point, but sometimes amniotomy is suggested to move labor along. The idea is that once the bag is no longer there, your baby's head will put more pressure on the cervix, encouraging it to open. There are no guarantees that this will work, but if your labor has truly stalled, breaking the waters may help avoid further interventions. However, if amniotomy is suggested just because the waters have yet to release on their own, patience may be the better option.

Intravenous Fluids (IV)

IV stands for *intravenous*, which means "inside a vein." A needle is used to place a thin plastic tube (catheter) into the vein. Whether or not you will have an IV during labor depends on hospital policy. Many hospitals routinely place an IV in laboring women, so if you prefer not to have one, be sure to ask your health-care provider beforehand. The IV not only provides hydration but also serves as a precaution in case an emergency arises, allowing easy access to a vein in case you should need medication quickly in labor.

Some health-care givers will offer you a heparin lock ("hep lock"), which means the needle is inserted into the vein but is not yet attached to tubing or IV fluids. A hep lock is more comfortable, since being connected to the tubing will limit your movements while you are laboring. This will keep the access to your vein ready, but will allow the IV tubes to be taken off so you can move around more easily.

Fetal Monitoring

Your baby's heart rate during labor is a good indicator of how well he is tolerating labor. When a baby's heart rate is in the normal range of 120 to 160 beats per minute, health-care providers can be reassured that the baby is receiving plenty of oxygen from the mother's bloodstream. Your health-care provider will be monitoring your baby's heart rate for abnormal variations, which could indicate decreased oxygen in his blood and tissues.

An electronic fetal monitor is an ultrasound device that uses straps to hold two monitors in place around your belly and records your baby's heart rate and your contractions on a continuous strip of paper. This allows your health-care provider to see how your baby is responding to contractions.

baby care tip

If you would rather not be connected to the fetal monitor for the early part of your labor (and you don't have a high-risk pregnancy), ask your health-care provider if you are a candidate for intermittent fetal monitoring. This means your health-care provider or nurse will put on and remove the monitor from time to time to check on your baby, and/or use a handheld ultrasound device called a Doppler, which was probably used during your prenatal visits. In early labor, the nurse will assess your contractions with his or her hands and listen to your baby's heart rate with the Doppler. Your provider will inform you when it is time for continuous fetal monitoring.

When more information about the baby's heart rate is needed, your health-care provider may recommend placing an internal electrode on your baby's scalp while you are still in labor. This is the most accurate method of obtaining the baby's heart rate.

Interventions in Delivery

Occasionally, late during the pushing stage, a baby is very close to being delivered but is not quite where he should be. This may be because the mother is exhausted and her pushing efforts are slowing down, or sometimes the baby shows signs (via the fetal monitor) that he needs to be delivered immediately. At some point your health-care provider may recommend using instruments such as forceps or a vacuum extractor to help expedite the delivery.

Although there is some risk with a so-called assisted delivery, if the tools are used properly they are very safe. Talk to your health-care provider prior to your delivery about the risks and benefits of forceps and vacuum extractors. You may want to ask about your health-care provider's statistics in using forceps and vacuums; these devices are typically used in less than 5 percent of births.

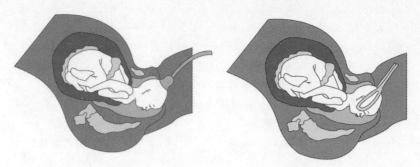

FIGURE 5-3: Vacuum-assisted and forceps delivery

Q. My baby had a vacuum-assisted delivery and now has a bruise on his head. Is he all right? How long will it take to go away?

A. Your baby just has some bruising and swelling as a result of the suction cup of the vacuum device. This swelling also results from the pressure of the cervix and birth canal on your baby's head (which can occur naturally as well). Both swelling and bruising will usually resolve within a day or two.

Q. I've been pushing for almost three hours and my doctor is recommending that we try an instrumental delivery with either forceps or vacuum. Why are they used and are they safe?

A. Forceps are never routinely used. In this case, you clearly need assistance because of pushing complications (you are exhausted, you cannot push due to anesthesia, or your baby's position is making it difficult to birth). The forceps will be placed around your baby's head and will help guide him through the vagina. They are a good choice when cesarean delivery is the only other option. (Just like the vacuum extractor, forceps are considered a safe delivery tool. Women should talk to their health-care provider about the risks during a prenatal visit.)

Q. When my friend gave birth she had something called an episiotomy, and it didn't sound pleasant. In what case would I need to have one? Are they routinely done?

A. An episiotomy is an incision made into the perineum to widen the vaginal opening to allow for birth. Some episiotomies are performed to avoid potential hard-to-repair perineal tears, but they are by no means routinely done. Other times an episiotomy may be performed if your baby is almost delivered but develops fetal distress. Pushing is hard on the mom, but babies can also get tired. If your baby is about to be delivered but is showing some signs that he is not tolerating the pushing anymore, your health-care provider may recommend an episiotomy to quickly deliver your baby.

Talk to your health-care provider during a prenatal visit about his or her episiotomy rate and the potential reasons for performing one. If you would rather tear naturally, which may or may not result in fewer stitches than an episiotomy, be sure to let your health-care provider know and include that in your birth plan. Keep in mind that you may not tear at all—another good reason for trying to avoid an episiotomy.

After reading this section, you may be concerned that labor and birth never occurs "normally." However, most healthy women have perfectly routine births with no complications or medical interventions. Being aware of these procedures is important so that when you are in labor, you will be more able to rationally discuss options with your provider if you run into any roadblocks. Always remember: unless you find yourself in a time-sensitive emergency during labor, take as much time as you need to discuss your options with your provider and, if you'd like, in private with your partner. There are often several nonmedical options you might want to try first. For example, if your labor has slowed down, instead of using Pitocin, ask your health-care provider if you can labor in the shower or on a birthing ball to help speed things up.

Cesarean Childbirth

The latest CDC statistics indicate that the current cesarean birth rate in the United States is approximately 30 percent (an average—some hospitals have lower rates and some higher rates), so it is possible that your baby may have to be delivered surgically if her health or yours is threatened. This procedure, during which your baby is removed from the uterus through an incision made in your abdomen, is known as a cesarean birth, cesarean delivery, or simply a C-section. Over the last ten years, cesarean birth rates in the United States have been on the rise. With one in every three births resulting in cesarean section, it is important that you have some information about the procedure so that you are prepared if your baby needs to be born this way. Understanding when and why this surgery may be necessary, how it is performed, and how to take care of yourself afterward will help to ensure that you have a positive birth experience.

Q. What kinds of circumstances might be reason for a cesarean birth?

A. Most cesareans are not actually done as emergency surgery; they are scheduled for previously identified health reasons, or when a cesarean simply becomes the best option during labor. There are a few unpredictable occurrences in pregnancy and labor that can prompt a last-minute C-section. Here are a few scenarios:

Prolapsed cord—On very rare occasion, the umbilical cord drops (or prolapses) into the vagina before the baby enters the birth canal. The baby's head might then compress the umbilical cord on its way out, which can decrease the amount of oxygen going to the baby.

Excessive bleeding—Most bleeding comes from the site of the placenta. If the placenta begins to separate from the uterine wall prematurely, this is called placental abruption. The seriousness of the bleeding depends on the degree of separation. A slight separation may result in light bleeding and mild cramping. When separation is slight to moderate, bed rest may be recommended to stop the bleeding. Treatment depends on the extent of the separation, but a severe separation is usually considered a medical emergency requiring immediate delivery of the baby.

Placenta previa—Placenta previa refers to the location where the placenta has attached to the uterus. Sometimes a placenta is low in the uterus, covering or partially covering the opening of the cervix. A low-lying placenta is common in early pregnancy, but it will usually move up as the pregnancy progresses and the uterus expands. The closer the placenta is to the cervix, the more likely it is to bleed. In some cases, the placenta will completely block the cervical opening and make a vaginal delivery impossible.

Failure to progress—Labor generally progresses more quickly once a woman is in the active stage (four or more centimeters dilated). Remember, in active labor the cervix is usually thinned out and begins to dilate more easily. However, there are times when labor may slow or stall regardless, and this is called failure to progress, sometimes resulting in a C-section.

Cephalopelvic disproportion (CPD)—If the baby's head is too large for the mother's pelvis, labor will slow down and a vaginal delivery may not be possible. Usually it is not that the baby's head is literally too large to fit, but rather that the position and angle of the head as it enters the pelvis affects the progress of labor.

Fetal distress—If the baby's heart rate pattern demonstrates a low level or lack of oxygen, health-care providers sometimes suggest delivering the baby via cesarean section.

Mother—If mother has a serious illness (such as heart disease or preeclampsia) or a herpes lesion or an infection, a cesarean birth may be suggested so as not to jeopardize her or the baby's health with a vaginal delivery.

Repeat cesarean—If mother has had a previous cesarean birth, health-care providers want to make sure she and the baby are both healthy and able to attempt a vaginal delivery. While the condition that led to a cesarean for one birth may not exist in a subsequent pregnancy, there are still a variety of reasons why a health-care provider may recommend a repeat cesarean.

Breech baby—When labor begins, most babies are head down. When a baby is not head down, a vaginal birth is not always possible. While there is always the possibility that a baby in a breech position will turn, by the end of the eighth month of pregnancy most babies do not have room to move around much anymore. Your health-care provider will determine the position of your baby by an abdominal or vaginal exam, sometimes supplemented by an ultrasound. Over 95 percent of babies are in the head down position, but some babies try to make their entry into the world with their feet or buttocks first. Whether or not you will be able to give birth vaginally in this case depends on your provider's policy, but you should know that most providers routinely perform a cesarean delivery for breech babies. If you are against such a policy for whatever reason, you may want to seek out a different health-care provider.

Q. What kind of preparation is needed for the surgery?

A. For a planned or non-emergency cesarean, the steps are typically as follows: You will be asked to sign a consent form, and then the nurse will start an IV if you don't already have one so that you may receive intravenous fluids. Next, you will be wheeled into the operating room (or walk in, depending on the situation). Once you are lying on the operating table, a blood pressure cuff will be put on your arm and monitors will be placed allowing the obstetrician and anesthesiologist to keep an eye on your vital signs (blood pressure, temperature, and respirations). In addition, an electrocardiogram (EKG) electrode will be placed on your chest to keep track of your heart rate.

A drape will be placed over your body so that only your abdomen is exposed. An additional drape will go across your chest so that your partner does not see the surgery. Around this time your birth partner, who will be prepped separately to enter the sterile environment, will be allowed in the room and usually will sit on a stool at the head of your bedside.

An anesthesiologist or nurse anesthetist will administer your anesthesia. The type of anesthesia used depends on the situation (see Pain Medication in Labor, page 117), but a spinal anesthesia is commonly administered through a needle into the spinal sac, relieving your lower body of any pain throughout the surgery. You may feel a tingling sensation at first, followed by numbing and a slight shortness of breath. However, if you have already labored with an epidural, many times simply adding anesthesia to the existing catheter will prepare you for the surgery.[14]

Once you are numb, a catheter will be placed in your bladder to keep it empty, and your abdomen will be washed off with an antiseptic solution in preparation for the surgery.

---

14   Carabuena and Kodali, "Anesthesia for Cesarean Delivery."

> ## baby care tip
>
> Sit back and relax—you won't feel any pain during a cesarean section, just sensations of movement around your abdomen and some pressure in your chest. And in no time your baby will be right there in the room with you!

Q. Who else will be in the room during the surgery?

A. A team of hospital staff will be involved in the procedure. Your doctor, or the doctor on call, and an assistant will perform the surgery. There will be a nurse in the room called the "circulator," who helps to keep everyone organized in the operating room, and a "scrub nurse," who hands the sterile instruments to the doctor. An anesthesiologist will be present throughout, as well as a pediatric team for your baby. The room may get very crowded, with a lot of hustle and bustle, but everyone will work together to safely deliver your baby. Don't let it bother you if you hear the team talk and even joke amongst themselves. As long as it is not an emergency C-section, the staff is usually very relaxed and calm.

Q. How long does it take to deliver the baby surgically?

A. Once the decision to perform a cesarean delivery is made, the staff moves very quickly. The baby is usually delivered within ten or fifteen minutes of the start of surgery, and it takes another thirty to forty-five minutes to close the incisions and complete the surgical procedure.

Q. When will I be able to hold my baby?

A. After your baby is born, the doctor or nurse suctions out the airways and clamps and cuts the cord. (Because the area around the abdominal incision must be kept clean, usually it is the doctor who cuts the cord in a C-section; a parent is not given the option.) At this time, the doctor will hold your baby up for you to see. While the doctor begins stitching the uterus and layers of muscle and tissue, your baby will be taken to a warming area and briefly examined by the pediatric staff. Once your baby is stable, which usually takes just a few minutes, the nurse can bundle him up in a blanket and hand him over to Dad or the birth partner.

When the repair is complete, the doctor will cover the incision with a large bandage. You should not be in any pain, but you may feel very sleepy, nauseated, or shaky. It is not a good idea to hold your baby until you are in the recovery room and feeling better. Some women can hold their babies within an hour, while others prefer waiting until they are more awake and alert. Expect that the blood pressure cuff will be left on and that your heart rate, respirations, temperature, and anesthesia level will be monitored every fifteen minutes or so for at least the first hour. If you feel up to it, ask your nurse or birth partner to place the baby close to you. There is no reason you cannot begin to hold or breastfeed the baby once you are considered stable by the medical staff.

baby care tip

There are two types of cesarean section incisions. The most common is a horizontal cut made in the lower segment of the abdomen, sometimes referred to as a bikini incision. The classical incision is a vertical cut made directly down the center of the abdomen. Because it is usually more difficult to repair, the classical incision is usually only performed if the baby or placenta are in unusual positions.

It can be challenging when something happens during the birth of your baby that is not part of your original vision for that day, such as a C-section or the use of medication. Keep in mind that it is normal to feel a wide range of emotions. On the one hand, you are excited to meet your baby and only want him to be safe; but on the other hand, you may feel disappointed. Anytime you go through something unexpected, you may need to mourn the loss of the experience you didn't get to have. Allow yourself to feel everything you need to in order to heal and move on.

Remember, at the end of the day the health of you and your baby are the most important things. No matter what kind of labor and birth you have, when you are finally holding your baby in your arms, the way in which she got there will likely seem far less important. If things don't go according to plan, try to replace any lingering negative feelings about the birth with positive ones about the wonderful days, months, and years ahead for you and your new family. While adjusting to life at home with a newborn may be challenging, each day will get easier and more joyful. As we will see in the next chapter, there are several ways to foster a smooth transition from your baby's delivery into your new role as a parent, and the hospital staff will be with you every step of the way for those first few postpartum recovery days.

· 6 ·

....

From Birth to Parenthood

....

After the many stages of pregnancy, labor, and birth, the moment your baby arrives you will be presented with yet another, whole new phase—parenthood! But, as you can probably guess, it won't be all cuddles with your baby and a wave goodbye to the hospital staff as you and your new family head home. This chapter will focus on the immediate postpartum experience, how you'll feel after your baby is born, and the hospital care you can expect to receive.

The postpartum period in labor and delivery, sometimes referred to as the "fourth stage of labor," will technically begin after the placenta is delivered and continue until you and your baby are stable enough to be transferred to your postpartum room. Although the postpartum stage can last for several hours, it may progress more slowly if the delivery was complicated or you had a cesarean birth.

During this immediate postpartum time as a new mother you'll experience rapid physical changes. Involution (the uterus returning to its nonpregnant state) will begin immediately after the placenta is delivered. You may feel very hungry and thirsty after birth, and the experience of labor and seeing your newborn for the first time will trigger the release of endorphins, stimulating adrenaline and a state of alertness in both you and your baby. Even though you may be exhausted, sleep will likely be several hours away! If possible, hold and cuddle your baby at your breast during this time while your body settles down, and savor the tremendous feeling of relief and joy that you and your partner will no doubt experience.

Q. I've heard it's a good idea to have my baby placed skin-to-skin on my chest after birth. Why?

A. As long as your baby is medically stable, holding her skin-to-skin has many benefits for both of you. Several studies have concluded that babies placed skin-to-skin are more likely to:

- Latch on to the breast and feed well
- Breastfeed longer
- Have normal skin temperature
- Have a normal heart rate and blood pressure
- Have normal blood sugar
- Cry less[15]

baby care tip

Partners: Mom will probably want to continue holding your baby after the birth, but it may still take some time before the birth is complete. Her health-care provider will still need to deliver the placenta and Mom may require some stitches to her perineum. While this is going on, your baby will be weighed, measured, diapered, and wrapped up in a warm blanket—now ready to be held and cuddled by you! This is a great time to find a comfortable place to sit and ask for the baby to be handed to you. Mom may need a few minutes to process the birth and refresh herself before holding the baby again. Take this time to sit and bond with your baby.

Q. I really wanted to have my baby placed right on my chest after delivery, but my health-care provider insisted that I place her on the warming bed until she stabilizes. Will I still be able to benefit from skin-to-skin later?

A. Absolutely—the positive effects of skin-to-skin are noted for several weeks following the birth. Remember that the primary concern of your health-care providers after the delivery is the well-being of you and your baby. Although they probably would like to be able to place your baby skin-to-skin immediately following the birth, your baby's

---

15   International Breastfeeding Centre, "The Importance of Skin-to-Skin Contact," ibconline.ca/information-sheets/the-importance-of-skin-to-skin-contact.

medical condition takes top priority. If your baby needs medical attention the best place for her is on the warming unit, where medical staff can care for her needs.

Q. I want to breastfeed my baby right way, but he's not interested in feeding right now. Should I be worried?

A. Don't be concerned if your baby is not particularly interested in feeding immediately after the delivery. Every baby is unique. Some are very eager to begin nursing and others are content just to hang out and relax. Your goal following the delivery is to enjoy this special time with your baby. Whether breastfeeding or just holding him close to you, your baby is getting to know his parents. I will discuss breastfeeding in greater detail in chapter 9.

Q. It took my baby a few seconds to take a breath after the delivery, and she did not cry right away. Is this normal?

A. The birth of your baby is a wondrous moment that you will always cherish. The first cries of a baby are not those of distress but a declaration of life. Your health care providers will be very happy to hear the loud cries of your baby, but not all babies cry immediately after the delivery. Some require some assistance from the pediatric team to stimulate and encourage those first breaths.

It's important to understand the amazing physical changes that occur during birth. In utero, your baby's lungs are filled with fluid and the oxygen supply is maintained through the placenta and the umbilical cord. After delivery, the fluid in the lungs is replaced with air. Your baby will begin to exchange oxygen for carbon dioxide and blood circulation to the lungs will begin.

A blood vessel called the ductus arteriosus is important during pregnancy to keep blood away from your baby's lungs. As fluid in the lungs is replaced by air, the increased oxygen levels will stimulate this blood vessel to begin closing. After the birth, your baby needs blood to circulate to the lungs. The ductus arteriosus is no longer needed and will usually close within a few days.

Q. I've heard that my baby will get an Apgar test. What does that mean?

A. The Apgar test reflects your baby's condition immediately following birth. It is given at one minute after delivery and then again five minutes later. The test is a tool for health-care providers to quickly evaluate your baby's condition and determine whether extra medical personnel should be called into the room to care for her.

The Apgar score will evaluate your baby based on five criteria. A score of zero to two is given to each criterion, so the highest total score a baby can achieve is ten. While the Apgar score is a good indicator of your baby's state, many babies simply require a few extra minutes after delivery to adjust to the world. In fact, many babies will have slightly blue hands and feet (I'll discuss your baby's appearance in more detail in the next chapter). This is all a normal part of the birthing process. Below is the American Academy of Pediatrics chart illustrating Apgar scoring.[16]

The Apgar Score

Sign	0	1	2
Skin color	Blue or Pale	Acrocyanotic	Completely pink
Heart rate	Absent	<100/minute	>100/minute
Reflex irritability	No response	Grimace	Cry or active withdrawal
Muscle tone	Limp	Some flexion	Active motion
Respiration	Absent	Weak cry; hypoventilation	Good, crying

7–10 points: Newborn is in excellent condition
5–7 points: Newborn is mildly depressed
Below 5 points: Newborn is severely depressed

---

16   American Academy of Pediatrics Committee on Fetus and Newborn and American College of Obstetricians and Gynecologists Committee on Obstetric Practice, "The Apgar Score," policy statement, *Pediatrics* 136, no. 4 (October 2015). pediatrics.aappublications.org/content/136/4/819.

Q. Why is my baby getting a vitamin K injection and antibiotic eye drops after birth?

A. Babies are routinely given eye drops after birth to prevent them from getting a serious eye infection from a sexually transmitted disease during passage through the birth canal. This is a public health measure and is usually done in the labor room shortly after birth. The drops don't appear to irritate babies' eyes, but some parents feel that they blur a baby's vision. If you want to delay the administration of eye ointment, talk to your health-care providers prior to the birth to discuss your options and hear their recommendations.

Vitamin K injections have been given to babies in the United States for the last fifty years. The vitamin K shot is recommended by the AAP and is standard newborn procedure in hospitals. In some states, the shot is mandated by law. It is given because some babies (about one in ten thousand, according to the AAP) are born with vitamin K deficiency, which can cause severe bleeding, possible brain hemorrhage, and even death.

If you would like to avoid any routine medication for your baby, be sure to discuss this choice with your health-care provider beforehand.

Q. I'm going to be a new dad soon, but I worry that I'll feel like I'm in everyone's way in the labor room. How can I bond with my baby amid all the people?

A. The delivery room is a busy place immediately after a baby is born. Don't worry too much whether or not you're "in the way"; you can begin bonding with your baby right away. If your baby is on the radiant warmer, go ahead and stand close to her, as the health-care team generally will not mind. If your baby is off the warmer and in stable condition, there is no reason you cannot hold and cuddle her. It's a good idea to sit in a comfortable chair and have the nurse bring your baby to you. Don't do too much walking around the hospital room with your newborn since it can be a very crowded place. If your hospital has a postpartum floor, you will soon be admitted into a much less crowded and more relaxing room. If you are staying in the same room, it will eventually become a lot less chaotic, so just hang tight, relax, and talk with your new baby. Remember, your baby has heard your voice throughout the pregnancy and is familiar with and comforted by its sound.

Physical Discomforts

In the first few hours postpartum, just try your best to rest. When you want to get up, don't jump out of bed right away—take your time, as you may experience dizziness or lightheadedness after the delivery. If you need to go to the bathroom, make sure there is someone in the room as you get up. Sitting on the side of the bed for a few minutes will help to stabilize your blood pressure, which should prevent the dizziness. If you still feel unsure about getting up, call your nurse, who will be more than happy to help you make it into the bathroom. You can shower as soon as you are walking around independently.

Q. I had an episiotomy and am very uncomfortable. What can I do for relief?

A. Episiotomies and vaginal tears do cause some discomfort in the perineum. You may get good relief with pain medication and ice packs for the first twenty-four hours, during which time they can reduce swelling in your bottom. It may feel good to continue icing for a few days, but another soothing remedy once the swelling has gone down is to use a warm sitz bath every few hours (your nurses will give you this portable device and show you how to use it). Use topical anesthetics and ointments from the hospital and do Kegel exercises to promote circulation and increase blood flow, which will help to heal the perineum. Finally, wash with warm water in the hospital squirt bottle instead of wiping after using the bathroom. The discomfort can last for several weeks, but you will gradually begin to heal and feel better.

Q. My bottom is very sore—will it hurt to go to the bathroom?

A. Many women experience an inability to urinate after a vaginal delivery. Drink lots of liquids. Pour warm water over your perineum as you're trying to urinate and keep the water running. These tricks usually work after a few attempts.

baby care tip

Take your pain medication as necessary for the first few days. The postpartum period in the hospital will be much more enjoyable if you are reasonably comfortable. Medications prescribed by your health-care provider are safe to take while breastfeeding. In addition to the medications, use ice packs on your perineum to help reduce swelling in the first twenty-four hours. (Ask your nurse where to get the ice packs, as this is something your partner can get for you.) In some hospitals, rubber gloves are filled with ice chips and tied in a knot. These work great but they do look very strange! If you're not sure about how to use the ice packs, ask your nurse to make sure you have proper placement—in fact, don't be afraid to ask the nurses if you're unsure about anything at all!

Q. Why am I so constipated? Is there anything I can do to ease my first postpartum bowel movement?

A. The combination of increased hormones, a decrease in activity, and relaxation of the bowel muscles conspire to bring on constipation. Many of the strong pain medications you may be using can also contribute to the problem.

Fear of having a bowel movement is common, especially if you have hemorrhoids or a lot of swelling in the area. It very well may take several days before you have a bowel movement. Here are a few ways to battle postpartum constipation:

- Drink lots of fluids; water is best, and prune juice often does the trick.
- Eat lots of fiber (fruits, veggies, whole wheat, bran, etc.).
- Take the Colace pill offered to you. If one does not work, ask for more—they are just stool softeners and are not harmful to you or your breastfed baby.
- Walk around, as this helps to "get things moving."

If you still feel very uncomfortable, you might need a suppository. Discuss this with your health-care provider and see what will be best for you. When you feel like you need to have a bowel movement (although this may not happen until you're home), kick visitors out of your room, bring a magazine to the bathroom if you have one, and try not to strain. Relax by closing your mouth and breathing downward.

baby care tip

After all the commotion, do yourself a favor and try to sleep when your baby does. Most babies are wide awake for a short time after birth and then fall into a deep sleep. This is a great time to get some rest after a tiring labor and birth. Ask your nurse to put a sign on the door that indicates you are sleeping.

Q. The nurse is pressing on my abdomen and it's uncomfortable. Why is she doing this?

A. Your nurse is performing a uterine massage to encourage uterine contractions. These contractions help to prevent excessive blood loss by closing off the blood vessels that previously supplied blood to the placenta. Assessing the top portion of the uterus (called the fundus) helps the nurse to determine the position and firmness of your uterus. Your health-care provider may also add Pitocin to your IV or give you an injection after delivery to encourage the uterus to contract.

After delivery, the uterus should feel hard and be approximately the size of a small cantaloupe. Within a few days, the uterus shrinks to about the size of a grapefruit and by week six it should be in its pre-pregnancy state (the size of a walnut, weighing about two ounces). Breastfeeding your baby will cause your body to release oxytocin, which will also help your uterus to contract.

baby care tip

Expect to have a nurse come in your room *at least* once every eight hours (hospital protocol is once every eight hours unless medically indicated) to check your blood pressure, heart rate, temperature, and vaginal bleeding, and check your fundus (top of the uterus) to make sure it is hard and contracted. This may be slightly uncomfortable.

The nurse will offer you pain medication to take if you're feeling uncomfortable, and it's perfectly safe to take this medication even if you are breastfeeding.

Q. Will I continue bleeding after the delivery?

A. Yes. You will continue to bleed for a couple of weeks at home. By day three postpartum the bleeding should slow down and may be similar to a menstrual flow. The amount of bleeding will diminish each day, and by the end of the first week the flow will be watery and pinkish in color. By the beginning of the second week, or between days ten and fourteen, your discharge will be yellowish-white in color. The amount tapers until about week three to four, when it usually stops.

This vaginal discharge and bleeding after birth—the drainage from your uterus—is called lochia. The amount of lochia varies from woman to woman. It is common to have a sudden gush of vaginal bleeding the first time you get up from your bed, as sometimes blood will pool in the vagina if you are lying down for several hours. When you stand to go to the bathroom, the blood may trickle down your leg or you may pass a few clots. As long as the bleeding stops after the clot has passed, it's usually fine, but tell your nurse if the bleeding continues or you soak through a pad in less than an hour. The nurse will monitor and evaluate your bleeding during the hospital stay.

Vaginal bleeding will have become less heavy by the time you are discharged from the hospital. If you notice an increase in bleeding after you are discharged, it is a sign for you to slow down. Put your feet up, have a drink of water, and make sure to note whether the bleeding slows afterward. If it does not, call your health-care provider. You should also call your health-care provider if you saturate a pad in less than an hour (soaking through the bottom of the pad) or you pass a clot larger than a quarter in size. Please note that clots are normal, and it is OK to have something smaller than a quarter for the first few days.

baby care tip

You may want to hold off before wearing your own undergarments after delivery, because you're likely to stain them. Most hospitals have disposable panties that can go into the trash after each use. Within a few days your bleeding will decrease, and you can safely begin wearing your own things again.

Q. I am so hungry and thirsty. Is it OK for me to eat after the delivery?

A. As long as your delivery is free of complications and you are medically stable, go ahead and eat. Labor is often compared to a marathon, and after childbirth your body will need energy to refuel. Immediately after labor, you can have your birth partner or nurse provide you with some fluids to quench your thirst. Water is always a good choice, but you may need something with some calories such as ginger ale or cranberry juice. When you are ready to eat, choose foods that are high in protein and carbohydrates to restore your energy. Many hospitals will offer a food tray after you deliver, or you can have your partner visit the hospital cafeteria to bring you a meal. It may not sound appealing now, but you wouldn't believe how many moms have told me that meal was the best of their lives after such a physical experience!

baby care tip

Partners: After the delivery is complete and things are calming down in the room, Mom will appreciate a thirst-quenching drink and perhaps even something to eat. Go ahead and get her what she wants. If your hospital floor does not provide snacks, make a trip to the cafeteria or a vending machine. It could be several hours before the hospital will send up a food tray. This is where those granola bars you packed from home will really come in handy for Mom!

Q. What happens in the cesarean recovery room?

A. After the surgery, you will stay in a recovery area for one to two hours until both you and baby are stable. You, your birth partner, and your baby will be in this area together. A nurse will frequently check your vital signs, such as respiration, pulse, and blood pressure. He or she will also check your abdomen and the incision where the surgery occurred, and may massage the uterus to make sure it is firmly contracted. Unfortunately, this will be uncomfortable—but brief! The IV and Foley catheter (to drain urine) will usually be left in place for twenty-four hours. Your nurse will show you techniques that will make moving in bed less painful.

Q. I can't wait to introduce the new baby to my family. Can they join us in the labor and delivery room?

A. Family members should not be encouraged to join you while you are still in the labor and delivery or recovery room. This is a time when nurses will be in the room frequently to monitor your vital signs, check your abdomen and vaginal bleeding, and check your perineum for swelling and possible bruising.

This is a great time for you and your partner to be alone, snuggle, and bond with your new baby. As previously mentioned, if you are stable, you can begin to breastfeed if you want to.

baby care tip

Enjoy the first hour or so with your new baby. It will be much easier for you to focus your attention on your baby without a room full of visitors. Your baby will be awake immediately after the delivery, a period sometimes referred to as the "quiet alert stage," when his eyes may be open and looking around; then he may go into a deep sleep for several hours. Use this waking time to get to know your baby, hold him, cuddle, and look into his eyes. Your baby will want to see you, too, and get to know you as well. You will have plenty of time later to visit with family and friends.

There will be a lot going on immediately after your baby is born, from the attentive hospital care both you and your baby will receive to the new emotions and bonding you and your partner will experience. And while there will inevitably be a recovery period, try not to fear the experience. You will be surrounded by health-care providers who share a common goal to support you and your new family in any way necessary. So when this time arrives, embrace it, relax, and cherish your new baby!

· 7 ·

Your Baby's Condition and Postpartum Hospital Procedures

Ten fingers, ten toes, what's next? As you first hold and examine your newborn, you will likely have a few questions about his appearance and the routine procedures and baby care that will follow those first moments. This chapter will give you an idea of what to expect when you first see your baby, describing many aspects of typical newborn appearance from head to toe. You've spent nine months thinking about your baby and have probably pictured yourself holding a perfect little angel. However, when the moment arrives and you are handed your baby, you'll realize that isn't exactly the case. Don't worry: no matter what, you will still think your baby is beautiful! But there may be some things you weren't prepared for, such as the cone-shaped head, the white coating on your baby's skin, or his swollen eyelids.

Your Baby's Condition

Q. I've seen plenty of plump newborn babies on TV shows and in magazines. Is this really what I can expect my newborn to look like?

A. No—most babies shown on TV and in the media are not newborns, but are closer to three months of age. They always seem to be visions of perfection with beautiful pink skin, perfectly shaped heads, and bodies as clean as can be. However, these images are not reality. Consider this: at the first moment you see your newborn, he will just have made his transition from a life immersed in amniotic fluid to dry air—via a rather small exit, if you birth vaginally!—and will also be going through some hormonal changes. These conditions may leave your baby with various skin blemishes or possibly a slightly misshapen head—all of which are normal and will likely resolve themselves eventually. Here are some of the most commonly seen newborn traits, some of which you can expect in your newborn after the delivery:

Skin—Immediately after delivery, your nurse will dry your baby off with a towel and probably place him on your chest. He will likely still be covered with vernix, a white waxy substance thought to protect the baby's skin from the amniotic fluid that surrounds it during the pregnancy. The amount of vernix decreases toward the end of pregnancy and most of it will be absorbed by the skin, eventually. Due to its powerful antibacterial proteins, there's really no need to wash it away.

Color—Your baby may have bluish hands and feet during the first few days after birth. But don't worry, this discoloration (referred to as acrocyanosis) is completely normal. It's just your baby's body regulating his temperature. Mittens and socks, while cute, won't really help. Hats are the way to go, as they help to heat your baby's core.

Milia—Milia look like tiny white pimples and may be found on and around your baby's nose because his sebaceous glands are not fully developed. Sebaceous glands are tiny glands in the skin that secrete an oily substance to keep the baby's skin lubricated. The best treatment is none at all—leave the skin alone and milia usually disappears within a few weeks.

Lanugo—Lanugo is soft and downy hair that covers your baby's skin in utero and typically begins to fall off during the third trimester of pregnancy. If your baby is born with lanugo it will likely be on his back, shoulders, and forehead, and you can expect for it to rub off due to friction of clothes and blankets within a month or so.

Stork bites—These are flat pink birthmarks occurring on the bridge of the nose, the eyelids, or the back of the neck due to the stretching of blood vessels. They may become redder when your baby cries or when there is a change in temperature. Stork bites on the face usually go away by age two, but those on the back of the neck may last into adulthood.

Café au lait spots—These are flat, oval-shaped, light brown patches of skin that typically do not fade or go away. If your child has six or more of these spots, mention it to your pediatrician because they could be associated with a medical condition called neurofibromatosis.

Strawberry hemangiomas—A result of dividing blood vessels, these are raised red birthmarks that may become markedly larger throughout your baby's first year but will typically fade away by the time he reaches school age. They are not painful and are usually not harmful.

Port-wine stain—This type of birthmark will look like red wine was splashed on your baby's skin. These marks start out light pink at birth but typically become darker with age. They can occur anywhere on the body but are commonly found on the face, neck, arms, and legs. Port-wine stains do not go away, but can eventually be treated with laser therapy if desired. If your baby has a port-wine stain on his face, be sure to get him evaluated by his pediatrician to make sure there are no other underlying medical issues.

Mongolian or cerulean spot—These marks are bluish-green in color and are usually found over the back and buttocks of babies that are of Native American, Asian, Hispanic, Mediterranean, and African-American descent (basically anybody with pigment in their skin!). They vary greatly in size and shape and typically fade away within a few years, but some persist.

Head shape—If you have a vaginal delivery, the pressure of the birth canal can cause molding, which makes your baby's head take on a cone shape. Your baby's skull is designed for this—it makes delivery easier and also gives you an excuse to put all those cute hats on the baby right away! Your baby's head will round back out in a few days. If you have a scheduled cesarean delivery, of course, your baby will not make the trip through the birth canal, therefore keeping his head a nice rounded shape. If your cesarean delivery occurs after an attempt at labor, your baby may still have some molding.

Fontanelles—Commonly known as "soft spots" on your baby's head, these are areas where the bones have not yet fused together. This allows for the rapid expansion of your baby's brain during the first year. Fontanelles are safe to touch and not as fragile as they look, although you should always be gentle when handling a newborn. By about eighteen months or so, your baby's skull bones will be fused together and the soft spots will disappear.

The smaller fontanelle is toward the back part of the head. The bones will fuse by two months and it will no longer be there. The larger fontanelle is more on top of the head, and it may not close until your baby is twelve to fourteen months old.

Swelling of breasts and/or genitals—Swelling of your baby's breasts or genitals is normal and happens because of exposure to maternal hormones. If you have a girl, she may also have a bloody vaginal discharge (called pseudomenses) as the hormone levels decrease in her body. Don't worry, the discharge does not need to be wiped away during diaper changes and it will go away during the first week.

This discharge should not be confused with uric acid crystals, which are brick-colored. If you find this substance in your baby's diaper, she may not be getting enough milk (uric acid crystals form in concentrated urine). Try to get your baby to eat more and the crystals will usually disappear within a few diaper changes. If they don't, contact your baby's pediatrician.

Five senses—By approximately the seventh month of pregnancy, your baby's senses have developed in utero and he is likely able to hear, see, taste, smell, and feel. However, some senses, such as vision, are not fully developed at birth and will take a few more months to mature. As loving parents, it is important that your baby's senses are stimulated (only to a certain extent during the first month of course!) so that they continue to get stronger.

Touch: Snuggle with your baby often throughout the day—he will be comforted and calmed by lying on your chest or by being rocked and cradled in your arms. He will also enjoy being lovingly stroked, caressed, and massaged.

Smell/Taste: Your baby will quickly learn to recognize your familiar scent. Although his taste buds won't be completely mature at birth, he will already prefer sweet tastes. Breast milk is very sweet and will taste very good to your baby, as will formula.

Hearing: During pregnancy your baby hears lots of muffled sounds such as voices, a dog barking, music, your heart beating, and even sounds of your digestion. Once born, your baby will be comforted by these familiar sounds, so go ahead and talk and sing to him right from the start! He will also likely calm when hearing soft rhythmic sounds—or even the whirring sounds of the hair dryer and vacuum cleaner!

Sight: The least developed of all senses at your baby's birth will be vision. Although he will be able to see, it will be several months until he develops 20/20 vision. At first he will best focus on objects between 8 and 12 inches from his face (the distance from your nipple to your face!). It is also thought that babies tend to prefer bold contrasting colors, such as black and white, to pale pastels during the first few weeks.

Newborn reflexes—Newborn reflexes are involuntary movements that can occur spontaneously or in response to a certain action. These reflexes actually help to identify normal nerve activity in a newborn. Here are some common newborn reflexes:

Rooting reflex: Stroke your baby's cheek and he will turn his head toward your finger and open his mouth to get ready to suck. This can be an indicator that your baby is hungry.

Grasp reflex: Place a finger in your baby's palm and he will grasp it tightly.

Moro reflex: This is also called the startle reflex because it usually occurs when a loud noise or movement startles your baby. Your baby will throw back his head and extend his arms and legs. It may look like he is reaching out to hold something.

Stepping reflex: Hold your baby in an upright position with your hands under his armpits and his feet touching a firm surface. He will move his legs as if he were walking.

Q. **What are newborn screening tests, and what other procedures should I be aware of?**

A. Newborn screening is the practice of testing newborns for over thirty potentially harmful disorders that are not usually detectable at birth. Most of these disorders are called "metabolic disorders" or "inborn errors of metabolism," and may include problems with a baby's use of nutrients to maintain healthy tissues or problems with hormones or blood. These programs are sometimes called "universal" screening programs because they are set up to test all babies. These conditions can affect a baby's normal development in many ways, and parents can pass along the relevant genes without even knowing they are carriers. Many hospitals give this blood test within the first forty-eight hours of a baby's life.

Hearing screen—Babies have their hearing tested before they leave the hospital. This is a very easy, quick, and painless test. If your baby fails the hearing test he will be referred for more detailed testing after discharge, but keep in mind that far more babies are referred than actually have hearing problems.

Jaundice test—Jaundice is a common condition in newborns and refers to the yellow color of a baby's skin and whites of the eyes, which is caused by excess bilirubin in the blood. Bilirubin is produced by the normal breakdown of red blood cells, and jaundice occurs when the bilirubin builds up faster than a baby's liver can break it down. High levels of bilirubin can cause brain damage in an infant, so if your baby's skin looks yellow, his bilirubin levels will be checked by either a blood test or by a skin sensor. If it is determined that your baby needs to be treated, he will likely receive phototherapy—special lights that help to break down the bilirubin in his blood. Your newborn will be placed under a large blue lamp that looks like an infant-sized tanning bed and will wear tiny "sunglasses" to protect his eyes. He'll wear only a diaper so that most of his skin is exposed to the therapeutic light. You can think of this as baby's first trip to the beach! (However, the light used is not ultraviolet—it is the blue portion of the visible light spectrum, so don't worry about UV exposure.) Your baby will also need to increase fluid intake, so even if you are breastfeeding, formula supplementation may be recommended. If you already have an established breast milk supply, you may be able to pump extra breast milk and use this for supplementation. Adequately feeding your baby helps prevent dehydration (which increases jaundice) and helps the gut eliminate the bilirubin that has already been processed by the liver.

Circumcision—If you have a boy, you will be faced with the decision of whether or not to circumcise him. Circumcision is the surgical removal of the skin known as the foreskin, which covers the head of the penis. It is primarily performed for cultural or religious reasons. Some circumcisions take place in the hospital before the baby is discharged, some occur after the baby is discharged, and some are performed during a religious ceremony.

The American Academy of Pediatrics policy statement on circumcision says that "the health benefits of newborn male circumcision outweigh the risks and that the procedure's benefits justify access to this procedure for families who choose it."[17] Because the AAP does not actually recommend routine circumcision, many parents wonder what they should do. Deciding whether or not to have this procedure done is something you should discuss with your partner before the baby is delivered. If the two of you are not sure, talk to your baby's pediatrician and your own health-care provider.

17   American Academy of Pediatrics, "Circumcision Policy Statement," *Pediatrics* 130, no. 3 (September 2012). pediatrics.aappublications.org/content/130/3/585.

Your Postpartum Stay in the Hospital

. . . .

The postpartum period begins typically one to two hours after you give birth. Once you have delivered your baby and are stable, you will leave your labor and delivery room and move into your postpartum room (if your hospital separates these functions; some do not). If you are moving rooms, expect to be transported in a wheelchair or perhaps even on a stretcher. Although you may feel like walking, your body will not be ready yet, so relax and enjoy the ride. Recovery from a cesarean delivery takes place in the recovery room, where your vital signs including temperature, pulse, and respirations will be monitored frequently. You will likely be in the recovery room for at least a few hours before you are stable enough to be transferred to a postpartum room.

baby care tip

Make sure to look around the delivery or recovery room before you leave so that nothing gets left behind. Common things that are easily forgotten are personal pillows, eyeglasses, cell phones and chargers, jewelry, and cameras!

Keep in mind that your wheelchair or stretcher will only accommodate a small overnight suitcase or bag, so pack light—the fewer personal items you have with you, the easier your transfer will be. Some couples come into the hospital with so much gear that getting to the postpartum room is quite an effort! There's no need to have your baby's car seat in the labor room, as is the case with most of your baby's things. When in doubt, leave belongings in the car until after the delivery. You can always return to the parking garage to retrieve them.

Your baby will also be with you at this time, but for safety reasons, hospital regulations will likely mandate that she travel in her own bassinet (hospital floors are slippery!). In fact, many hospitals insist that babies be in their bassinets whenever moving in the hall—which means no walking in the hospital corridors with your baby in your arms.

Your partner will be with you throughout this time and will help load up and transfer your personal belongings. But remember, his job will also be to wheel the bassinet to the new postpartum room, leaving his hands pretty full!

baby care tip

If you are planning on bringing your own pillow, make sure the case is anything but white. Hospital pillows are white so you'll want your pillows to stand out. It can be a bit chaotic when you are transferring or leaving a room, and many times white pillows are easily overlooked and forgotten.

When you arrive on the postpartum floor you will be greeted by your postpartum nurse, who will be wearing proper identification. Most of the hospital staff that work on maternity floors have special identification on their badges and many wear pink ID bands. Your labor and delivery nurse will hand your care over to your postpartum nurse. When doing this handoff both nurses will check ID bands on you and your baby, and very likely your partner as well. Checking ID bands is done constantly in the hospital to ensure correct identity of all babies. Although occasionally you hear about a baby mix-up in the news, it is actually a very rare occurrence. Some hospitals have sensors on all babies that sound an alarm if a baby is ever taken off the floor without permission. Do not remove these tags until you are discharged.

If you have formed a special bond with your labor nurse, it can be a bit emotional to start over with a new nurse. But know that postpartum nurses are specifically trained to assist you during these first few days with your baby, so within a few hours you will probably feel very comfortable with your new nurse. However, she may have several other new moms to care for, so it is expected that you and your partner will take the lead in caring for your baby at this point. This will help you gain confidence as new parents.

To cut costs and to promote breastfeeding, many hospitals are phasing out newborn nurseries, and most modern birth centers never had them to begin with. Understandably, some argue that it just adds more unfair pressure on moms to breastfeed and does not necessarily add support for them. Others point out that such "cost-saving measures" won't translate into lower co-pays for patients. Having worked as a nurse and lactation consultant in Boston maternity hospitals for over a decade, I can attest that there are indeed benefits of shifting away from the longtime practice of nurseries. For the entire pregnancy, you and your baby are one. It doesn't make much sense to break up that unity so soon after birth, unless medically necessary. This should be a time for skin-to-skin with mom (and dad or partner). It should be a time for getting used to feeding and learning how to care for your baby. In fact, many mothers aren't even able to fully rest or relax when their newborn is in another room full of other babies. Many have recalled to me the anxiety they felt hearing cries of an infant in another room and worrying it was *their* little one. And there you have it—the mommy guilt begins!

If you're at all concerned about not having the option of a nursery after you have your baby, simply bring up your concerns with your health-care provider or the hospital administration ahead of time to make sure you understand their guidelines. If you're not happy with their nursery and rooming-in policies, simply find a new hospital that is more in line with your needs.

If you find yourself not feeling well while you're *in* the hospital postpartum, speak with your nurse. If it relates to your well-being, she should be able to work something out. You can also ask friends and family to come help out while you get some rest, too.

Q. What will I be expected to learn during the postpartum hospital stay?

A. The nurse will show you how to change and swaddle your baby, and assist you with feedings. If you are breastfeeding, your nurse will spend extra time with you to make sure that you get off to a good start. The nurse will also tell you about any classes that may be offered by your hospital or videos/DVDs that may be available for you to watch. Take advantage of the classes and videos offered—they are designed to provide you with the latest in infant care. Try to limit visitors or have them come after the classes so you are able to participate.

baby care tip

Use your time in the hospital to learn as much as you can about taking care of your baby. Listen carefully to what your nurses have to say—and, since you will be very tired, ask to hear the information repeated if necessary! Talk to them about any questions or concerns you have—this is the time for you to tap into valuable expertise and get comfortable with handling your newborn. You should also try to limit your visitors so that you can have time to rest. Your friends and family will be excited to meet your little one, but they will understand that you also need this time to bond.

Q. I was told to wait a few hours before having visitors. What will I be doing during this time?

A. The first hour or two on the postpartum floor is not the best time for visitors. Visitors should remain in the waiting areas until the nurse completes your admission, and sometimes this takes a few hours. You will be hearing a lot of information from your nurse at this time. Try to listen and focus on what your nurse is explaining. She will orient you to your room, tell you about the postpartum unit, and give you special telephone numbers so people can call you. She will also explain hospital procedures and protocols for taking care of your baby, including feeding instructions and diaper care. She will demonstrate how to use the bulb syringe (which some parents find intimidating, but which is really very simple) to clear your baby's nasal passages if necessary. Your nurse will also show you where all of the baby supplies are stored in your room—diapers, wipes, ointment, T-shirts, blankets, and so on.

Partners are encouraged to participate by handling diaper changes and recording their times on paper. It's also very helpful for partners to keep track of feedings—whether you're using a bottle or breastfeeding, tracking the times your baby eats is very important for the first few days.

If you are recovering from a cesarean birth, your birth partner may be doing most of the baby care for the first two to three days. It's good to discuss this possibility beforehand. Of course, it's fine to ask the nurse to show you how to change the baby's first diaper, but after that it is up to you to care for your little one. Hands-on experience is the best, and before long you will be an expert! Parents who are hands-on in the hospital come home with so much more confidence in taking care of their babies.

Q. Should I keep my baby in the nursery during the first night?

A. Only if medically indicated; otherwise, it is up to you to decide whether to keep your baby with you or send him to the nursery for a few hours. The decision is very personal and there is no right or wrong choice. Many women feel exhausted and benefit from a period of uninterrupted sleep. Bringing your baby into the nursery does not automatically mean he will get a bottle of formula and a pacifier, but it is up to you to let the nursery staff know what your wishes are. If you are breastfeeding and choose to send your baby to the nursery, make sure you tell the nurses not to give your baby a bottle, and realize that you may only get a two- to three-hour stretch of sleep before it is time to feed again.

If you wake up in the middle of the night and want your baby, you can call and ask that he be brought to you, or you can get up and take a walk—which, again, is good for you—and check on the baby. If you have been up several hours with your baby in your room and then want him to go to the nursery, you can call or bring him there yourself. There are no strict rules and regulations about this. But while nursery care is there if you need it, rooming-in with your baby is highly recommended and allows you to spend this special time together as a new family.

Q. I would like to keep my baby in the nursery at night and have the nurse give her a bottle so I can get a good night's sleep. Will this interfere with breastfeeding?

A. That depends—every baby is different. Some babies take a bottle of formula during the night and go back to the breast without difficulty. Other babies take a bottle and then get very frustrated at the breast because bottles are so much easier for them. Formula flows out of a bottle very quickly while breast milk takes longer, at least when you first start breastfeeding. Breastfed babies need a bit more patience. Sometimes I see babies latch easily to the breast but then become frustrated if the milk does not flow quickly enough. Ultimately, while it is important that you get as much sleep and rest as possible, it is also very important, if you want to breastfeed, that you do so very often in the first few days to build up your supply and get yourself and your baby used to the process.

I will discuss whether to give your breastfed baby a bottle more thoroughly in chapter 9, but in general, keeping your baby at the breast as much as possible is a good idea. Of course, there are several medical reasons why your baby might need a formula supplement and that is absolutely fine. (Babies who have lost more than 10 percent of their birth weight or babies who are jaundiced will usually need formula supplementation.) The first priority is to have a healthy baby. The hospital nurses or a lactation consultant will help if your baby is having problems staying latched. Ask your health-care provider to supply you with a list of lactation resources available in your community.

baby care tip

If you are planning to breastfeed your baby but you or your health-care provider would like to supplement with formula, try to use a method other than a bottle, such as a cup or a syringe feed. Your nurse can show you how this is done. That way your baby is less likely to get confused next time he feeds at the breast.

Recovering from a Cesarean Section

Q. I'm having a scheduled C-section. What can I expect in the postpartum period?

A. You will likely be very tired and groggy immediately after the surgery. Some moms who feel like this actually sleep for a few hours. As mentioned previously, you will stay in the recovery area until both you and baby are stable and then a nurse will transport you via stretcher to your postpartum room. Your nurse will orient you to your room and make you feel comfortable in your new bed, but will also urge you to get out of bed and take a walk. At first you may only be able to take a few steps, and then you'll gradually increase your activity level. Expect to get up within eight to twenty-four hours of the surgery. Your nurse will be with you the first time you get out of bed to make sure you are ready and stable to walk.

baby care tip

It is very important to start moving around as soon as possible after your C-section, as this will help you to feel better sooner. The idea of walking right after surgery may seem crazy at first, but don't underestimate yourself! Walking helps to speed up the process of moving gas through the intestines. Try to get out of bed and move around as soon as your nurse gives you the OK. Take your time when getting out of bed—go slowly and sit at the side of your bed for a few minutes before you come to a complete stand. Your first walk may be to the bathroom and back, and that's fine; increase your activity each day. By your second day, you will probably be able to walk the halls, and by day three you can impress your visitors with a walking tour of the maternity unit.

Take your prescribed pain medications. Most are compatible with breastfeeding. Everybody has different thresholds for pain, so if the medication that you receive isn't working, discuss this with the nurse—you may need to take the medication at shorter intervals or need something stronger for the first few days to get past the pain. Along the same lines, talk with your nurse if you feel a particular medication may be a bit too strong.

Q. I have sharp abdominal pains that radiate all the way to my shoulders. What can I do for relief?

A. Abdominal gas is usually present after any abdominal surgery, including a cesarean delivery. Intestinal activity stops during the surgery, and this can result in an accumulation of gas. The reason your shoulder hurts is that the air gets trapped inside you and moves up toward the shoulder area; this is called transferred gas pain. Physical movement, such as walking, deep breathing, and sitting in a rocking chair, may alleviate the discomfort of gas buildup caused by the surgery. Talk to your health-care provider about a pain reliever.

Q. Will I be able to eat after cesarean delivery?

A. Procedures vary by health-care provider and hospital, but if your condition is stable you can usually expect to start eating solid foods between four and eight hours after delivery. Start off slow with some liquids and then gradually move to some easily digestible foods. Your nurse will listen to your bowel sounds to make sure your intestines are functioning again and you are ready to begin eating.

baby care tip

Keep your diet on the bland side for a few days. Stay away from greasy burgers, pizza, and fries, especially if you are having gas pain. Peppermint tea is great to help relieve bloating and gas. To help alleviate gas, try drinking hot or warm drinks such as tea, and avoid carbonated beverages.

Q. Will I have a vaginal discharge after a cesarean delivery?

A. Yes, you will have lochia just as if you delivered vaginally, though perhaps a bit less. It will be a bright red bloody discharge for the first few days, and then it will change to brown and then to a yellowish color. You will probably have to wear a sanitary pad for a few weeks.

Q. What can I expect to feel like at home the week after a cesarean?

A. You will still be sore and have pain from your incision, but you will most likely be taking pain medication for the discomfort. Every day you will notice a decrease in pain and your need for medication will eventually diminish. You will be eating, drinking, walking around, and gradually resuming many activities. You will probably not feel up to driving for a few weeks, and you will also tend to avoid the stairs. In order to avoid slowing down your recovery, it is a good idea to avoid strenuous activity: no lifting anything heavier than your baby for the first two weeks. That also means no housework!

Your doctor will most likely want to see you at about two weeks postpartum. This is a good time to discuss your activity level and ask what level of exercise is appropriate for you. By your sixth week postpartum, you can usually resume all of your previous activities.

Q. Can I try to have a vaginal birth with my next baby, after this cesarean birth?

A. Yes. This is called a VBAC, which stands for "vaginal birth after cesarean." Your health-care provider will talk to you about a trial of labor for your next birth. If all goes well, labor will end with the vaginal birth of your baby. If complications arise during your trial of labor, a repeat cesarean delivery will have to be performed.

The Birth Partner

Most hospitals want to make both parents' stay as comfortable as possible. Partners are encouraged to spend the night and will have some sort of cot or chair bed to sleep in (although this might not always be the case in double rooms). Extra pillows and blankets will be provided by the hospital.

Some hospitals provide meals for partners while some do not; you may want to find out about your hospital's meal policy beforehand. Toiletries for partners are usually not supplied by the hospital either, but most gift shops carry emergency toiletries, such as razors and shaving cream, and pain relievers.

baby care tip

Partners, make sure you pack a small bag of items including water, a light snack, personal care products, ibuprofen or some type of over-the-counter pain reliever. The night of your baby's birth could be a long one, so having these things in your room may be much needed!

Q. I'm a new dad. This is my third day in the hospital and I'm exhausted. It would be great to go home tonight and get a good night's sleep so I'm rested tomorrow when I bring my wife and baby home, but I don't want my wife to have to be alone with the baby. What should I do?

A. You are not alone—this is a common question many partners have. Your wife will not be alone during the night. The nursing staff is available round the clock to answer any question or concern that she has. Whatever assistance she may need, whether feeding the baby or changing a soiled diaper, the hospital staff is on call to help her all the way. If you need to catch up on sleep, tell your wife how you feel. Most likely she will be happy to have a rested husband on hand to help out a lot during the next few days.

Q. My wife has been very emotional since the birth of our baby a few days ago. She seems to cry for no reason at all. What can I do or say to help her?

A. The so-called baby blues occur during the first few days and weeks after birth. Baby blues are normal, and they tend to go away in a few weeks without medication. The rapid fluctuation in hormones after birth, mixed with fatigue, can make many moms weepy and teary at certain times during the day. The best thing you can do for your wife is to be caring and supportive: Tell her that you love her and provide her with lots of encouragement. This is a temporary state and she will very likely be feeling like herself again soon.

baby care tip

Mom, if your tears and feelings of sadness continue for more than two weeks then you may have postpartum depression (PPD), which is a bit more complicated than simply baby blues. You may need therapy, a support group, or antidepressant medication for a while. No one knows the exact cause of this depression, but it is thought to be the result of chemical changes in the brain brought on by the rapid fluctuation of hormones after birth. I will address PPD in more detail in chapter 10.

Discharge from the Hospital

Once your stay at the hospital has come to an end (if you have any questions about what day you'll be discharged, just go ahead and ask), your nurse will go over the discharge protocol with you. She will check and record all of your vitals one more time, ensure that your bleeding is stable, and, if you've had stitches put in, check that everything is

healing properly. She will also likely go over basic baby care and feeding schedules with you one more time, to make sure you feel prepared
as you return home with your newborn.

Q. **I am being discharged from the hospital today, but the
nursery wants to keep my baby here until they get the results of
some tests for infection. Is there another room I can stay in for the
night, or do I have to go home without my baby?**

A. The idea of leaving the hospital without your baby can be fright-
ening, but many parents end up having to do this for various reasons,
including a baby born prematurely, a baby who has elevated bilirubin
levels (is jaundiced), or, in your case, a baby with signs of infection.
Unfortunately you cannot keep your own hospital room during your
infant's extended stay, as your hospital will need to make room for the
next batch of postpartum mothers.

Ask your nurse if there are any special rooms reserved for circumstances like yours. Such a room may not be private or even have a bed,
but it will be a place in which you can camp out until doctors give your
little one the OK to head home. You can always work out a schedule
with your partner so that at least one of you is at the hospital while the
other sleeps more comfortably at home. If there really isn't anywhere
you can stay at the hospital, there's absolutely no reason to feel guilty
about heading home for the night and returning in the morning to be
with your baby. She will be in great hands and you can get some rest.

Your postpartum time at the hospital will be spent bonding with your
new baby and receiving lots of guidance from your health-care providers on the ins and outs of baby care and recovery. I recall working
with one new mom who seemed tense in her first postpartum days due
to a few breastfeeding complications. I reassured her that she was
doing a great job and let her know I was there if she wanted to talk
about anything at all. After I reached out to her in this way, she really
opened up about how she was feeling and was visibly more relaxed
and happy as a result. That's what your postpartum health-care providers are there for: not only to tend to you and your baby's physical
care needs, but to educate you, listen to you, and answer your questions—to *support* you. Take advantage of this experience and never

hesitate to speak up about anything you're feeling. Whether you need a little emotional support, seek more information about something, or want to ask the nurse manager to reassign that nurse who puts you a bit on edge, your health-care providers want to help you in any way they can so you can leave the hospital feeling confident and excited to take on your new role as a mom.

· 8 ·

Parenting a Premature Baby

Every week that your baby spends growing inside your uterus counts. While some women may joke about wanting their little one to make an appearance early—especially toward the end of a long, exhausting pregnancy—they know keeping the "bun in the oven" full term is important. Unfortunately, though, sometimes babies *do* arrive before their lungs, brain, and other systems are fully developed. In fact, one in ten babies were born prematurely in the United States in 2014, Centers for Disease Control research found.[18] But this chapter shouldn't scare or worry you. With modern medical care and a lot of love and support, preemies are capable of developing into strong, healthy, and happy children—I've witnessed this throughout my career more times than I can count! This chapter is meant to give you an idea of what you can expect if you find yourself delivering early.

So what's considered "early"? The American College of Obstetricians and Gynecologists (ACOG) states it is "when birth occurs between 20 and 37 weeks of pregnancy." Preterm birth can occur for a host of reasons, yet often the cause is unknown. Risk factors include:

- Carrying multiple babies
- Cervical insufficiency or uterus complications
- Having had a prior preterm birth

---

18   Centers for Disease Control and Prevention, "Preterm Birth," cdc.gov/reproductivehealth/maternalinfanthealth/pretermbirth.htm.

- Maternal smoking, drugs, or alcohol abuse during pregnancy
- Maternal infection or illness

Being aware of and addressing such risks with your provider early on in your prenatal care may help decrease your chances of delivering preterm. In addition, "listening" to your body can help you identify when you may be experiencing preterm labor. Signs include cramping, tightening of your belly, pelvic pressure, a leak or gush of fluid (water breaking), and changes in vaginal discharge. If you experience any of these or a general feeling that something's not right, contact your provider immediately to determine the next steps.

Despite the known risk factors for having a preterm infant, sometimes the reason babies come early is unknown, and it's certainly no one's "fault." And although feeling guilty is a very common, normal response, it's important for moms to stay positive and try not to spend time and emotional energy on self-blame. The best plan of action is to quickly get rid of any ideas of what your birth experience would have been like, accept where you're at, rely on your medical team, and move ahead—there will be time for reflection at a later date. Furthermore, it's crucial that parents make sure to take good care of *themselves*, because nurturing a preterm infant is a long road and often challenging. By getting enough sleep, eating well, and accepting help and support from others, parents will be at their best to care for their infant(s).

Preterm Birth Complications

According to the ACOG, "The risk of health problems is greatest for babies born before 34 weeks of pregnancy. But babies born between 34 weeks of pregnancy and 37 weeks of pregnancy also are at risk."[19] Because premature babies are born before they are physically ready to leave the womb, they often have health problems and are given extra medical attention and assistance immediately after delivery. The degree to which your baby may or may not have these issues most often depends on the gestational age (number of weeks into pregnancy) of the baby at birth. Some of these include:

> **Apnea and bradycardia**—Apnea is a prolonged disruption of a regular breathing pattern (to stop breathing for more than twenty

---

19 American College of Obstetricians and Gynecologists, "Preterm (Premature) Labor and Birth," acog.org/Patients/FAQs/Preterm-Premature-Labor-and-Birth.

seconds or so), while bradycardia is the slowing of the heart rate. These two can occur as a result of an undeveloped nervous system that is common in preterm infants. Medicines, oxygen, and ventilation are common treatments.[20]

Chronic lung disease (CLD)—CLD is a term for respiratory problems that can occur long-term as a result of undeveloped lungs upon birth, and the damage sometimes caused by medical treatments administered to such fragile lungs. Blood tests and X-rays can help diagnose CLD, and treatments may include ventilation, oxygen, and medications such as antibiotics, steroids, and/or diuretics.[21]

Feeding issues—Preterm babies are often not developed enough coordinate effective sucking, swallowing, and breathing for feeding by breast or bottle. Intravenous fluids or special feeding tubes that go from the mouth or the nose to the stomach are often methods used to provide necessary nutrition and hydration.[22]

Jaundice—Because a preterm baby's liver is not yet fully developed, it may not be able to remove enough bilirubin, the substance produced when red blood cells break down, causing a yellowing of the skin and whites of the eyes. It can be diagnosed through physical exam and blood tests, and the primary treatment is phototherapy (absorption of light through the skin), although a special type of blood transfusion may be warranted in some cases because too much bilirubin can cause injury to the brain.[23]

Neurologic issues—The preterm baby's brain and neurologic systems will continue to develop after birth, but the early delivery may have some effects on brain development and function, such as risk of bleeding and delayed development.

Respiratory distress syndrome (RDS)—RDS is a disease that occurs when undeveloped lungs lack surfactant, a substance that helps keep lungs open and filled with air. The medical team will perform

---

20   Department of Pediatrics, Emory University School of Medicine, "Apnea and Bradycardia," pediatrics.emory.edu/divisions/neonatology/parent_info3.html.

21   Stanford Children's Health, "Chronic Lung Disease," stanfordchildrens.org/en/topic/default?id=chronic-lung-disease-90-P02348.

22   Medline Plus, "Neonatal Weight Gain and Nutrition," medlineplus.gov/ency/article/007302.htm.

23   Medline Plus, "Newborn Jaundice," medlineplus.gov/ency/article/001559.htm.

tests to determine if an infant has RDS and will take steps to treat accordingly, which may include providing a careful flow of oxygen, using a ventilator to help the baby breathe, or administering surfactant into the airways.[24]

Retinopathy of prematurity (ROP)—Because normal retinal development depends on a full-term pregnancy, the retina of infants born earlier than 31 weeks have not received enough oxygen and nutrients to complete the process. This can stop development and cause abnormally enlarged blood vessels, which, if left untreated, can cause retinal detachment, vision loss, or impairment. Treatments for advanced ROP include laser therapy, cryotherapy, or surgical procedures.[25]

In summary, the breadth and severity of complications will differ from baby to baby. Also, preterm infants have a weaker immune system, which makes them more susceptible to infection.

Q. I feel so overwhelmed and am not sure I understand everything that's going on with my baby's health. How can I possibly absorb everything?

A. Whatever complications may arise, *never* hesitate to ask—and re-ask—the medical team questions about your baby's condition, medications, and treatment options. Discuss decisions with your partner and do your best to trust and take comfort in the care your little one is receiving.

Preterm Baby Appearance and Condition

Media, television, and movies don't often portray preterm babies, so as a society we're not accustomed to seeing the sometimes drastic differences when compared to a full-term baby. Because of that, it can be quite shocking at first to take in the sight of a preterm infant. Appearance and size will of course vary depending on gestational age, but common characteristics of preterm babies include:

---

24 Medline Plus, "Neonatal Respiratory Distress Syndrome," medlineplus.gov/ency/article/001563.htm.

25 National Eye Institute, "Facts About Retinopathy of Prematurity (ROP)," nei.nih.gov/health/rop/rop.

- Large head in relation to body
- Less muscle mass
- Minimal fat
- Sharper facial features
- Thinner and more transparent skin
- Visibly labored breathing
- Yellow skin

baby care tip

Following all hospital procedures to minimize risk is critical until the infant has had time to mature and develop.

The Hospital Experience

One of the difficult aspects of having a preterm infant is that you don't get that initial joy of holding and spending time with your newborn baby. Because the medical team needs to assess and treat the infant right away, preterm babies usually go straight to the special care nursery (SCN) or neonatal intensive care unit (NICU) before you're able to see or touch your baby. She may also be cared for in a different location than you are, and it's not easy to move around the hospital to see your new baby when you are recuperating yourself. Rest assured, however, that the medical team will provide the best possible care for your preemie, even if it means moving the baby to another hospital for more specialized care.

A baby's condition upon birth, and progress thereafter, dictates in what section of the hospital she is cared for. NICUs have several levels: The level II NICU is for babies born closer to full term (typically between 32 and 37 weeks) and with relatively minimal complications. Level III is for infants born severely premature or with life-threatening complications that require specialized expertise and technology. A NICU is staffed by a neonatologist (a pediatrician with advanced medical training in the care of premature or very ill infants), nurses and nurse practitioners, and respiratory therapists, and the "team" may also include a nutritionist, a lactation consultant, a social worker, and a feeding specialist.

Like all areas of a hospital, the SCN and NICU have their own unique equipment. And while all the beeping, buzzing, and occasional high-pitched alarms of the NICU often become a parent's "background music," at first it can all be overwhelming—understandably so. It's frankly *really* scary to see such a small human being hooked up to so many wires, tubes, and machines. But if you do find yourself in this position, try to remember that those procedures and medical devices— along with the care teams monitoring them—are working together toward the optimal recovery, development, and health of your baby. Some of the most commonly seen NICU equipment includes:

Bili lights (phototherapy)—These fluorescent blue or green lights are placed next to or shine onto the baby's skin to help treat jaundice (reduce high bilirubin levels). While under bili lights, baby must wear eye patches to protect his eyes.

Blood pressure monitor—Similar in function to a blood pressure monitor you see in a doctor's office, the NICU has a special cuff that goes around an infant's limb and regularly monitors and records blood pressure.

FIGURE 8-1: A preterm baby in an incubator

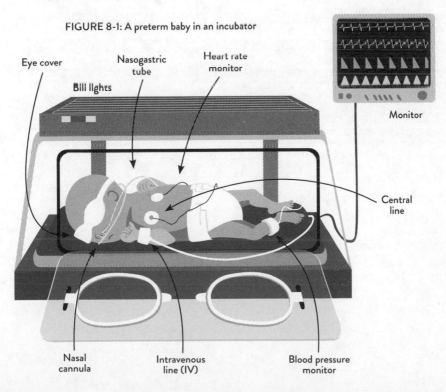

Eye cover

Bili lights

Nasogastric tube

Heart rate monitor

Monitor

Central line

Nasal cannula

Intravenous line (IV)

Blood pressure monitor

Cardiopulmonary monitor—This machine makes sure baby's breathing is regular and his heart rate is at a safe level. Small monitoring pads are placed on baby's chest and information is fed to a machine that beeps if his breathing isn't as it should be.

Central line—Much like an umbilical catheter, a central line is a small tube that is placed in a large blood vessel (usually in the chest, neck, or groin), which can be used by the care team to administer medications or take blood samples.

Continuous positive airway pressure (CPAP)—Preterm infants who require pressurized air, but can still breathe on their own, receive it through small tubes connected from the nose or windpipe to a ventilator.

Incubator—Incubators are a warm, quiet, relatively womb-like haven for premature infants to help protect their underdeveloped systems. They are transparent, plastic, covered "beds" that allow parents and caregivers to see and touch baby without fully exposing him to the air and atmosphere of the NICU.

Intravenous line—An intravenous line is a short, soft catheter inserted through the skin into a vein, usually in the hand or foot, that can provide the baby with fluids, medication, and nutrition.

Mechanical ventilator—Sometimes premature infants are unable to breathe on their own and require help from a mechanical ventilator. This machine provides adequately warm and humid oxygen to baby through a small tube inserted in his nose or throat/windpipe until his lungs are ready to perform the job independently.

Nasal cannula (nasal prongs)—These help provide baby with oxygen via small plastic tubes in his nose.

Pulse oximeter—A pulse oximeter is a small light sensor attached to baby with a piece of soft tape that's typically wrapped around his hand or foot. It's used to detect the level of oxygen in the blood.

Radiant warmer—Radiant warmers may be used in place of an incubator as a heat source for an infant who either is a bit more unstable or requires constant hands-on care.

Umbilical catheter—The catheter (a very small tube) is inserted into a blood vessel at the location of the cut umbilical cord through which the care team can provide medicines, nutrition, and fluid, as well as draw and give blood. This can also help monitor baby's blood pressure during the first ten days after birth. Although it looks and sounds uncomfortable, think of it as an effective and painless way to provide baby with thorough treatment and monitoring.

Length of Stay

Your baby's condition and gestational age will determine where and how long the hospital stay will be. Some late-preterm infants respond well to treatments and medications and can be discharged within just a few days or weeks, while others may need to stay for three to four months or more. It's important not to try to rush this process—it takes time for such a fragile little body's premature systems to develop, and for baby to become strong enough to breathe and eat independently. That said, it's not an easy experience for any family to go through, either emotionally or logistically. Here are a few things you can do to make the best of things:

- Get acquainted. Take the time to get to know your baby's care team and the NICU staff, and be present for scheduled rounds (updates on your baby's status). Developing these relationships will give you peace of mind, especially when you are not able to be by your baby's side.
- As you sing to and snuggle with your baby through the NICU days and nights, be sure to reach out to friends and family for support. You will need as much support as you can get in order to recharge and stay strong for your fighting newborn.
- Go home. You're going to spend *a lot* of time at the hospital nurturing your baby to health. But once you're discharged from the hospital yourself after birth, it's important to regularly get a good night's sleep and recharge with healthy home-cooked meals. Your baby will be well cared for (and resting up, too!) while you're away for a bit.
- If you or your partner work outside of the home, discuss your options for medical leave with your employer. Prepare yourselves for a long-term recovery process and the financial stress that may accompany it.

You and your partner will notice a certain routine developing while your baby is in the NICU, including regular check-ins from the medical team to discuss progress and next steps. For medically stable infants, one of the most crucial parts of that routine will often be regular "kangaroo care"—laying diapered baby on his parent's bare chest to allow skin-to-skin contact. While parents of full-term babies are typically *encouraged* to take part in this practice, it's critical for parents of preterm babies to do so, if they are allowed. Kangaroo care relaxes infants, warms them naturally with body heat, helps regulate breathing, promotes breastfeeding, and leads to more solid sleep. It can also help strengthen the bond between baby and parents, reduce maternal stress, and boost breast milk production. That said, providing skin-to-skin kangaroo care may be an intimidating experience, especially at first. As discussed, preterm babies often have tubes and wires attached to them to help with feeding and monitoring and to administer medication. This can understandably make some parents scared to hold their fragile-looking baby, feeling they may accidentally disrupt the urgent medical care their baby is receiving. But just as with anything new and scary, it *will* get easier over time as it becomes part of a daily routine. Once you see how much your baby seems to love kangaroo

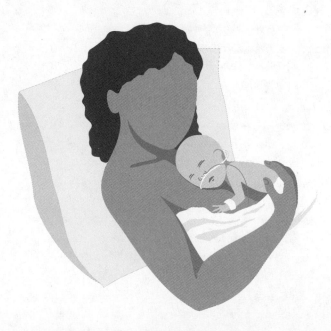

FIGURE 8-2: Woman providing kangaroo care to baby in the NICU

care and being softly spoken to, you'll treasure that time. Reaching out to your medical care team with questions every step of the way will also help you feel more at ease.

Feeding a Preterm Baby

Proper nutrition intake is essential to a preterm baby's development and health progress. A nutritionist works with parents and the medical team to determine the amount and frequency of feedings, and when it comes to what a preterm baby consumes, the "breast is best" slogan is particularly sound. The American Academy of Pediatrics policy states, "The potent benefits of human milk are such that all preterm infants should receive human milk. Milk from the infant's own mother, fresh or previously frozen, should be the primary diet, and it should be fortified appropriately for the infant born weighing less than 1.5 kg [3.3 pounds]. If the mother's milk is unavailable despite significant lactation support, pasteurized donor milk should be used."[26] Indeed, most hospitals have access to milk banks that can help supply your premature baby with donor milk!

The AAP cites significantly lower rates of sepsis (a serious immune response to bacterial infection) and necrotizing enterocolitis (a damaging intestinal disease that often warrants surgery) with preterm infants who consume breast milk, as well as the ability to take in complete nutritious feedings earlier on. Before preterm infants are able to feed at the breast, mothers typically pump every two to three hours and baby is fed through a tube. Pumping and storing *can* be time consuming, but it's well worth it for baby's health in the short and long term, as the AAP states, "The benefits of feeding human milk to preterm infants are realized not only in the NICU but also in the fewer hospital readmissions for illness in the 3 years after hospital discharge."

Women who experience pumping or milk supply problems should discuss and coordinate human milk donor programs with the NICU care team. If parents cannot or choose not to use breast milk, however, specialty formulas for the premature baby's gut will be introduced.

---

26   American Academy of Pediatrics, "Breastfeeding and the Use of Human Milk," *Pediatrics* 129, no. 3 (March 2012). www2.aap.org/breastfeeding/files/pdf/Breastfeeding2012ExecSum .pdf.

Hospital Visitors

Because preterm babies are so vulnerable and need time with their *parents* most of all, it's important that visitors are kept to a minimum. Discuss visitation policies with your NICU nurse, as policies vary from hospital to hospital. Generally, one or two siblings are allowed in at a time and must have proof of up-to-date vaccinations. Visitation of siblings under the age of two is usually not recommended, and there may be certain times of the year when children of any age are not allowed. All visitors must be healthy—no one with colds, fevers, or other symptoms should come to the hospital. A visitor's pass will likely be issued by the hospital, and before entering the NICU, all visitors must wash their hands thoroughly with soap and warm water. Once inside, all visitors should maintain the calm, quiet environment preterm infants need, and although it may be hard *not* to look around at the other patients in the NICU, it's important that everyone focuses only on the baby they're there to support.

baby care tip

Celebrate the small steps! Every test passed and every ounce gained matters. Yes, having a premature baby who is struggling to develop can be a rollercoaster ride and sometimes presents difficult challenges, but having positive energy will help lift you and your partner up, particularly during the more difficult days.

Taking Baby Home

When a preterm baby is medically stable and showing promising signs of healthy growth and weight gain, the care team determines readiness for discharge. The NICU team commonly:

- Provides a written update to baby's pediatrician, as well as recommended next steps, weight gain, check-up frequency, and so on.

- Prepares parents on what to expect and how to care for baby at home. Parents may be given a notebook or instructions that highlight important knowledge, such as how to mix a higher-calorie formula, track diaper output, administer medications/treatments, and so on.

- Conducts a car seat test. Babies born before 37 weeks are at increased risk of oxygen desaturation (a drop in oxygen level in the blood). Baby is placed in a standard car seat for a prolonged period while the care team monitors her breathing, heart rate, and oxygen levels. If the baby passes the test, it's safe to use the car seat upon discharge. If not, baby will likely need to use a car bed until a follow-up test is passed in a few days or a week.

- Sets up a visiting nurse agency to come to the home if baby meets criteria. The visiting nurse will check on the health of mom and baby, answer questions, provide support for breast- or bottle-feeding and wound care, perform labs if the doctor has ordered any, and, if needed, coordinate community services for the family. If a visit is ordered, the nurse will call you on her own to schedule a visit. The visits are typically less than an hour.

- Refers baby to a local early intervention program, if baby meets criteria. Early intervention is mandated by the U.S. government to assess and provide services from birth to age three, particularly for babies who are born prematurely and may need extra services to reach developmental milestones.

- Helps coordinate infant CPR training for parents and other potential caregivers, if necessary.

Although you may have been dreaming of bringing your baby home, it's completely normal to feel anxious when it actually happens. Why *wouldn't* it, when you're used to having a top-notch medical team around to constantly monitor your baby and round-the-clock resources to run questions by? It can be tough to go from that to trusting a sole pediatrician your baby sees once a week. And if baby is discharged along with medications or other devices you need to be responsible for, it can add even more stress. But just understand that this *will* be a transition, and you should seek out a local support group of NICU parents—they will listen, understand exactly how you're feeling, and may help quell concerns. The "normal" challenges any parent faces with a newborn are there of course, but then there are also challenges specific to caring for preterm babies, including:

The guilt—Feelings of guilt over the time *not* spent by baby's side while in the NICU can haunt parents. It can make them feel like they need to make up for that once they're home. But while premature babies *do* need special care and attention, they don't need to be held all day long or to be picked up at every sound they make. It's a parent's job to help establish healthy sleeping, soothing, and feeding routines, which can be tough if you don't get rid of the guilt and carve out some time for you and your partner to reconnect.

Corrected/adjusted age—You may have heard a first-time parent refer to their baby's age in weeks or months (well into the toddler years, even!). With a preterm baby, however, it's more nuanced than just counting days on the calendar. There's the chronological "actual age," which is counted from the date of birth. But "corrected age" adjusts for a baby's prematurity. According to the University of Nebraska Medical Center, "When a baby is born early, his brain and the rest of his neurological system have not developed or matured to the same degree as a baby born at term."[27] Thus, for the first year of your baby's life, health-care providers will usually evaluate your premature baby on both chronologic age and corrected age. To calculate baby's corrected age, simply subtract the number of weeks premature from baby's actual age.

Weight gain and development—Parents of full-term babies often compare their kids to others of the same age, from height and weight to when they begin crawling or climbing. But due to the reality of corrected age, preterm babies may take a while to "catch up" in terms of growth and development—and that's OK. You may choose to let those playgroup conversations go or explain the concept of corrected age to those who may not know. Either way, utilize the help of primary care and subspecialty physicians and early intervention programs wherever possible to continue on a positive path for your little one.

---

27   University of Nebraska Medical Center, "Understanding Corrected Age," unmc.edu/media/mmi/jackson/TIPS-Intro/Understanding_Corrected_Age.pdf.

Q. How do I cope with my first nights and days home from the NICU?

A. It's OK to be fearful! As long as you've discussed any concerns with your baby's care team or pediatrician and have a plan in place should an issue arise, you can sit back, be confident in the skills you've learned, and enjoy your baby. Find the few minutes each day to care for yourself—reading or catching up on social media while you pump, or any activity that helps you relax. But note, while it's normal to feel "baby blues," anxiety, or guilt here and there, if you feel it's overwhelming you, discuss those feelings with your health-care provider immediately.

Welcoming Multiples

Imagine. After weeks of settling into the idea of having your first baby—dreaming about who he or she will be—you hear the words or see on the ultrasound monitor that things aren't exactly what they seemed. That you're actually carrying *more than one* sweet baby! It happens. In fact, the latest figures from the Centers for Disease Control show that the multiples rate in the U.S. is at an all-time high, with twins accounting for 33.9 per 1,000 live births and triplets 113.5 per 100,000 live births.[28]

The rise in multiples births may be caused by several factors; the greatest is the trend toward delayed childbearing. More and more women are opting to complete higher education and establish careers before starting a family. After the age of thirty or so, women tend to have more than one egg per cycle (increasing twin chances) as well as higher levels of a follicle-stimulating hormone, which is tied to fraternal twin births. The use of fertility drugs and advances in artificial reproductive therapy (ART) contribute as well. Given the relative prevalence, throughout the rest of the chapter I address some of the questions parents tend to have when it comes to caring for multiples, including how to navigate their common preterm birth status.

---

28   Centers for Disease Control and Prevention, "Multiple Births," cdc.gov/nchs/fastats/multiple.htm (from "Births: Final Data for 2014," *National Vital Statistics Reports* 64, no. 12, December 23, 2015).

Q. My sister just had fraternal twins. Does that mean I am more likely to as well?

A. Yes, compared to the general public, if you have a mother or sister who has had fraternal twins, you may be twice as likely to have fraternal twins yourself![29]

Let's begin with twin basics. According to the National Library of Medicine, identical twins "occur when a single egg cell is fertilized by a single sperm cell," while "fraternal twins occur when two egg cells are each fertilized by a different sperm cell in the same menstrual cycle."[30] Identical twins look so similar because they share the same DNA. Fraternal twins, on the other hand, are genetically like regular siblings in that they only partially share the same DNA.

Whether fraternal or identical, though, twins tend to share an incredible connection that many parents do their best to nurture. The commonly held belief is that since multiples occupy the same small space for so long, it's comforting and beneficial for them to continue spending significant side-by-side time once born. While there are benefits to this, it's important to remember that what multiples need above all else is to have their basic and emotional needs met by their *parents* on an individual level. In the flurry of feedings and sleep deprivation, it can be hard to keep that at the top of your mind. There's even a tendency to attribute certain characteristics to babies based on factors out of their control (such as who was born first!), and those labels often carry on as they grow. But being conscious from the very beginning that each of your little ones is indeed their own person who needs regular one-on-one attention and love to develop a sense of self may help avoid any twin frustrations long-term.[31]

Support

Upon learning you're pregnant with twins or triplets, seriously consider joining a local multiples club. There you'll find a great sense of camaraderie and support from parents who have already gone through

---

29   U.S. National Library of Medicine, "Is the Probability of Having Twins Determined by Genetics?" ghr.nlm.nih.gov/primer/traits/twins.

30   Ibid.

31   See the Web site of twin expert Joan A. Friedman for more information on twins: joanafriedmanphd.com.

the "shock and awe" of having multiples. They'll provide advice, warm words, and an understanding ear. Membership usually includes monthly meetings where you can meet other parents in person—both expecting and seasoned. Some mothers stay in these clubs even when their "babies" become adults! Most clubs these days have Web sites with resources and discussion boards, or active Facebook groups. Others offer age-specific multiples playgroups, and even family outings. Many also have tag sales, where members can shop first for great bargains. But even if you don't join during pregnancy, you can always consider it at any point postpartum or as your babies grow.

Carrying Multiples

Statistics have shown approximately 60 percent of twins are born preterm, with triplets at closer to 90 percent. For this reason, along with an increased risk of low birth weight, preeclampsia, and gestational diabetes, your pregnancy may be considered "high risk." This designation is not meant to cause you alarm but to ensure that you and your babies are monitored appropriately. You'll likely need to check in with your health-care provider more frequently than a typical singleton pregnancy, and you'll want to be sure to follow all of the recommendations made at each prenatal visit. Don't hesitate to contact your health-care provider—day or night—with any concerns you may have, or if you are experiencing preterm labor at any point during your pregnancy. While bed rest has historically been prescribed in an effort to prevent preterm labor, the ACOG's current position is that it is not effective.[32] If preterm labor is noticed early, however, your provider may take advantage of medications and treatments that help postpone labor and best prepare your babies for an impending premature birth.

Maternal nutrition and adequate weight gain are critical for multiples pregnancies, as they promote higher birth weight and development. According to the latest Institute of Medicine (IOM) guidelines, a woman with a normal pre-pregnancy body mass index should ideally gain between 37 and 54 pounds during a twin pregnancy, while a healthy triplet pregnancy weight gain would be approximately 50

32   American College of Obstetricians and Gynecologists, "Physical Activity and Exercise During Pregnancy and the Postpartum Period," Committee Opinion no. 650 (December 2015). acog.org.

to 60 pounds or more depending on your pre-pregnancy weight.[33] How can you stay on track? Consider healthy eating your full-time job. You'll need to nourish your growing babies with high-calorie, vitamin-dense foods in frequent small quantities (which can help with morning sickness nausea). You'll want to try to consume approximately 300 extra calories per day, per baby. Discuss these specifics with your health-care provider and consider consulting a nutritionist as well, to help you establish and stick with a solid pregnancy nutrition plan.

Bringing Home Your Babies

Unfortunately, sometimes with preterm multiples at different stages of development, one baby can be discharged from the hospital before the other(s). It can be really difficult to juggle caring for two or more infants in two different locations, so naturally parents tend to experience feelings of immense guilt. Communicating with your partner about how you're both feeling and coming up with a hospital/home schedule will help get you through this period. Be sure to enlist family members and close friends to help "cover shifts" as well, until your babies are home together.

As covered earlier in this chapter, when you do finally have everyone home from the hospital, it can be both a relief and overwhelming all at once. All parents experience sleep deprivation to some degree, but parents of multiples experience it exponentially—there *are* more babies to care for, after all! One baby may fill the proverbial "night owl" role, while the other may sleep for hours-long stretches after their nighttime feeding. You never know how it'll go. Work with your partner to feed and soothe consistently and establish a routine. Instituting a schedule will take time, though, so try to be patient and stick with it.

Here's a look at a sample routine that may help you get an idea of what a typical day might look like once you settle in with your multiples at home. Keep in mind, this is simply a general guide intended to help you out. Something like this may or may not work for you. If it doesn't, don't worry—you'll establish one that does.

---

33   K. M. Rasmussen, P. M. Catalano, and A. L. Yatkine, "New Guidelines for Weight Gain During Pregnancy: What Obstetricians/Gynecologists Should Know," *Current Opinion in Obstetrics and Gynecology* 21, no. 6 (December 2009): 521–26.

Sample Routine for Stay-at-Home Breastfeeding Mom and Working Dad with Four- to Eight-Week-Old Twins

TIME	TASK	SUGGESTIONS
5:00 AM	Breastfeed	Use twin breastfeeding pillow to breastfeed both babies simultaneously.
5:40 AM	Change/ Sleep	Partner burps and changes babies, swaddles them, and puts them back down to sleep so you can get some more sleep and he can get ready for work.
7:30 AM	Breastfeed	Use twin breastfeeding pillow to breastfeed both babies simultaneously, taking care to alternate the breasts each used for the previous feeding. Partner helps burp, change diapers, and get babies dressed before work.
8:15 AM	Play/Pump	Lie on the floor with both babies and talk to them during brief tummy time. Put them in bouncy seats or swings and pump any leftover milk so your partner can help feed in the evening. Eat breakfast while the twins are occupied in their seats.
9:30 AM	Change/ Breastfeed	Use twin breastfeeding pillow to feed both babies simultaneously, taking care to alternate the breasts each used for the previous feeding.
10:00 AM	Sleep	Swaddle babies and put them down to sleep.
10:15 AM	Downtime	While you have two free hands, use this time to prep lunch and dinner, do a load of laundry, shower, and have a snack so you're ready to attack the rest of the day.

TIME	TASK	SUGGESTIONS
11:30 PM	Change/Play	Change the babies to make sure they're awake for their upcoming feeding. Sing and talk to them as you do so.
12:00 PM	Breastfeed	Set yourself up on the sofa with your twin breastfeeding pillow (and a tall glass of water) to breastfeed your babies.
12:30 PM	Sleep	Swaddle both babies and put them down to sleep.
12:45 PM	Lunch/ Downtime	Make sure you eat a healthy lunch (you burn approximately a thousand calories per day just nursing!). This is also a good time to have visitors. Arrange for them to bring meals or stop at the grocery store on their way over.
2:30 PM	Change/ Breastfeed	Play with your babies as you change their diapers to make sure they're awake for the feeding. Return to your "nest" on the sofa (with a glass of water) to feed both babies.
3:15 PM	Play/Walk	Call a friend to go for a walk with you and the babies so you all can get some fresh air if weather permits. Otherwise, put your babies back on their tummies and interact with them face-to-face.
5:30 PM	Change/ Breastfeed	Change the babies and settle down to breastfeed both of them before dinner.
6:00 PM	Sleep	Partner helps swaddle the babies and put them down for a nap.

TIME	TASK	SUGGESTIONS
6:15 PM	Dinner/ Downtime	Eat a healthy dinner and enjoy downtime with your partner. You can both, of course, do a few chores that may need addressing.
8:00 PM	Bath/Change	Give babies a bath and dress them in pajamas.
8:30 PM	Breastfeeding	Feed both babies and let your partner help burp them.
9:00 PM	Sleep	Read the babies a story and swaddle them. Put them down to sleep.
11:30 PM	Change/ Breastfeed	Breastfeed one baby at a time in bed, with your partner's help burping and changing diapers.
12:00 AM	Sleep	Swaddle the babies and put them back down for a long stretch of sleep.
4:30 AM	Change/ Breastfeed/ Sleep	Change if necessary, then feed babies one at a time lying in bed, or your partner can feed one bottle of expressed milk. Swaddle and put the babies back down to sleep after minimal burping.

baby care tip

Keep several baby "stations" around your house, especially if you have more than one level! You will definitely appreciate having all your supplies close by, no matter where you are, including wipes, diapers, creams, drool cloths, swaddling blankets, extra outfits, and snacks for you!

Visitors

Understandably, friends and family will want to come help out once your babies are home (and meet and snuggle with them, too, of course!). And I certainly encourage taking them up on those offers as they relate to things such as shoveling the driveway or dropping off groceries, supplies, or homemade meals—as long as they're convenient for *you*. But as previously mentioned, for the first few days and weeks after birth or at home, keeping visitors to a minimum for *any* baby—particularly preterm—is a good idea. This not only reduces the likelihood of bringing unwanted sicknesses into your babies' environment, but gives you, your partner, and your little ones low-key time to settle in, establish a routine, and bond with one another. It also allows you time to learn and build confidence in your new roles as parents. That may sound strange, but parenting newborn twins "with an audience," so to speak, isn't as easy as it may seem. Yes, most will be well meaning, and some will offer valuable support. But chances are there are a few you'd frankly rather not hear "advice" from so early on—some who have a tendency of putting you or your partner on edge. There's no need to put yourselves in that situation so early. Discuss this with your partner during your pregnancy and decide who you *would* be willing to have come meet your babies earlier rather than later. Start laying the foundation and relaying your wishes to friends and family. Getting off to a positive start with your infants can't be redone. So do what you can to establish the scenario *you* will comfortable with.

As you do start accepting visitors (who *aren't* sick, of course!), ask that they wash their hands with soap and warm water before holding the babies. I know this can feel awkward, like you're being overprotective, but I assure you, you're not! The American Academy of Pediatrics recommends it. If it feels too awkward to have the conversation, send a text beforehand, place a friendly reminder on the front door, or designate another person to relay the message. Strategically placed bottles of hand soap can also be a good subtle reminder that hygiene is a priority around your little ones.

Most visitors will ask if there's anything they can do to help—others won't. Either way, don't be shy, and tell them! If there's laundry in the dryer, ask them to grab it and fold. If the dishwasher needs unloading, let them know. Are you hungry? Ask for a snack and a glass of water. Your babies will need *you* most of all, so be sure to communicate ways that friends and family can assist you in doing your number one job.

Feeding Multiples

Feeding preterm multiples is a challenge—one that sometimes may feel insurmountable but that you *can* do and that *will* get easier. To make sure each baby is taking in enough nutrition and growing sufficiently, there will be regular weight checks while in the hospital. This may need to continue for a bit when your babies are discharged—whether through frequent visits to the pediatrician or in your own home through a visiting nurse agency. You will be introduced to special growth charts, depending on your babies' gestational age at birth, to guide you.

If your multiples are born prematurely, it is imperative that they are woken up for feeds, and fed as often as instructed by your babies' medical team. A three-hour feeding schedule is typical, and with two babies it can be trial and error to determine which feeding plan works best for your family. Some parents alternate feedings (one rests while the other parent feeds both babies). Some do feedings together—each parent feeds one baby. As the babies grow and develop, your preferred feeding methods will likely change. Don't be afraid to experiment. What works best one month may not work best the next month!

Breastfeeding

In an ideal world, all babies would latch easily, breastfeed on schedule, and sleep perfectly well. But the truth is, each is an individual with his own needs and preferences, so embrace whatever routines and positions work best for you. Because preterm babies' systems are not yet fully developed, they typically have trouble latching. Pumping and bottle-feeding is your best bet until they reach the time frame of their "due date," after which they will start to develop the skill of latching and staying on the breast for feedings. Regular kangaroo care from the start can help promote this milestone. Discussing different techniques with a lactation consultant early on while they are still in the hospital can help as well. They will give you lots of suggestions for how to get your babies latched on, how to nurse both at once or one at a time, how to supplement if necessary, and more. When you make the transition home with your babies, however, be sure to discuss next steps with the lactation consultant and make contact with La Leche League, an international nonprofit that promotes breastfeeding, which will provide local support group information.

Buying or renting a good pump may help with breastfeeding your multiples. You may find it difficult to produce enough milk for two babies, so pumping frequently right from the beginning will help increase your milk supply. In addition, you may want to give your babies pumped milk from a bottle sometimes—either because you need to add to what they are getting from the breast or because your partner or other caregiver would like to help feed them.

There are a number of nursing pillows on the market, but I suggest you purchase one made especially for twins. These pillows tend to be thicker, more supportive, and designed in a way that angles the babies toward your body. You can also use them for bottle-feeding. What's more, they usually come with a detachable pillow that supports your lower back. While the babies are small and you're getting the hang of feeding them, ask your partner or other support person to hand you the pillows so you can get them into place and then ask for the babies one at a time so you can get them into a successful position.

Once feeding is established, you may find that you want to place one baby to breast each feeding, breastfeed both at the same time, or alternate breast and bottle every other feed. *You* need to decide what is best for you—and of course your babies will have a say, too! Remember, the job of a newborn is to put on weight, so your babies will nurse frequently and sleep most of the time between feedings. As often as you can, be sure to sleep when they do, even though that will usually be just two to three hours at a time. You need to take care of yourself in order to be able to take care of your babies.

Bathing

For safety reasons, and to give you and each baby one-on-one bonding time, I recommend giving baths to your babies separately—alternating days, perhaps. Preemie babies have less fat than those born full term, so keeping baby warm is important before, during, and after bath time. Heating up the bathroom ahead of time can help keep baby calm and relaxed for bath time.

You don't need to bathe your babies every day—two to three times a week is fine. In between, just use a warm washcloth to keep their faces and neck crevices clean, along with any other areas that may need washing. You will find more detailed instructions on giving baby a bath in chapter 10's Baby Care Basics section.

Q. How on earth do I get out of the house with twins?

A. I know the idea of it sounds crazy at first, but preparation (and practice!) is key. A backpack may be easier for baby supplies than the standard diaper bag. Consider keeping extra supplies stocked in every car you use—it helps with the last-minute forgotten items! Don't forget to restock any of the extra supply bags frequently and keep a stroller in the car with you, even if you are going short distances. You never know when you might have to evacuate the car with your multiples.

You will find that multiples garner *much* attention. You may want to have some ready answers to frequently asked questions—Are they twins? Did you have them naturally? Are they identical? While it can be frustrating, know that most people are generally interested in and in awe of multiples. Having your partner, a family member, or a friend with you the first few times you go out with your babies may help as you build up your confidence.

For a parent of multiples, it's easy to feel a bit isolated, and preparing for and taking trips outside of the home can be exhausting. Please know that this is normal. After a month or two, push yourself a bit to spend time out of the home to gain confidence. Every trip you'll learn something new and you'll feel like you conquered a mountain!

DOS AND DON'TS WITH MULTIPLES

- Do take one baby out and about and leave the other(s) at home with another caregiver regularly.
- Do utilize one of the many meal or grocery delivery services.
- Do utilize diaper delivery services and online shopping for supplies.
- Don't feel you always need to answer the phone or texts. Get to them when you can.
- Don't compare yourself to others. Raising multiples is a truly unique challenge and each parent has their own path.
- Do hire or accept help caring for your babies if you're feeling overwhelmed. There's no shame in it, and a little baby-free time or solid sleep will do wonders for you (and your babies!).
- Do contact your care provider immediately if you experience prolonged feelings of sadness or irritability.

Baby Essentials

When it comes to things your babies need, let the supply list in chapter 1 guide you. They will each need their own car seat and crib or bassinet, and it's never a bad idea to have a stroller that fits everyone. Plenty of comfortable cotton Onesies-style bodysuits and sleepers are a must—quantities of which really depend on how often you want to do laundry! You'll also need plenty of extra diapers, wipes, and feeding supplies. If you choose to use a baby monitor, you may want to purchase an extra camera to ensure clear views of each sleeping baby.

You really don't need to buy (or register) for double of everything, but it does help to have a few safe lounging spots (swing, bouncy seat, play mat) where you can put one baby down while you're feeding the other(s). Slings and carriers can be a great resource as well, and while there are some made for carrying twins simultaneously, for your body's sake, I recommend wearing one baby at a time.

In short, when it comes to baby gear, keep in mind that your babies don't need to be having the same experience at all times—in fact, it's important that they each have their *own* experiences and maintain their own special bond with you.

Visit sites like multiplesofamerica.org and raisingmultiples.org for more helpful information on caring for and raising multiples.

PART III

Breastfeeding Your Baby

· 9 ·

Bring Your Lactation Nurse Home

One of the most important choices you will make as a new parent is whether or not to breastfeed your newborn. While the benefits of breastfeeding are widely known, many women give up on nursing because they are overwhelmed and confused about how best to make it work for them and their baby. This chapter will highlight the various health benefits of breastfeeding for you and your baby, and discuss what you can expect from the experience. I will provide a series of recommendations and support options to make breastfeeding effective and comfortable.

Although it seems natural that you and your baby would intuitively breastfeed well together, many times this is not the case. Yes, most babies are instinctual suckers, but they may not be instinctual latchers. The art of breastfeeding needs to be learned. Even if you have close friends or family who have nursed their babies (or have had trouble breastfeeding), we as women do not tend to absorb much detail about breastfeeding until it becomes our own reality. Be prepared for the possibility that you may have a few obstacles to overcome for the first few days after delivery and that you may experience some frustration and disappointment. Of course, most babies who start off with a few challenges eventually end up breastfeeding successfully. If this is not your first baby, remember that every baby is different and each breastfeeding experience will vary. Understanding how breastfeeding works and how to manage potential difficulties that can occur is important for success and will ultimately make a huge difference in your breast-feeding experience.

As a certified lactation consultant working in several Boston hospitals, I have come across many different types of breastfeeding issues. One new mom I cared for had a breast reduction ten years before she gave birth, but she was always told that she would be able to fully breastfeed regardless. She was very intent on breastfeeding and wanted very badly for it to work. But after her baby was born her milk supply was not enough to feed her baby. When he kept losing weight the pediatrician recommended supplementation with formula. She felt like she was a failure and deeply regretted her decision to have the breast surgery. Together we established a plan that would both allow her to breastfeed her baby and make sure he got enough nutrition by also supplementing with formula. She started using a breast pump and her milk supply gradually increased, but never to the point of sustaining her infant. However, within a few weeks we had developed a great feeding system and she felt happy knowing she was contributing what she was able to. Throughout this chapter, I will share real-life breastfeeding situations like this one and common nursing questions that new parents have during their hospital stay and the early weeks at home. Most breastfeeding issues have a simple solution, while others may take several weeks to address and get back on track—either way, you'll need a little bit of nursing knowledge and a lot of patience! I will explain the many benefits of breastfeeding for baby and mom, the anatomy and physiology of the breast, and how breastfeeding works. We will delve into colostrum and the composition of milk, including foremilk and hindmilk, and discuss engorgement, expressing milk, and breast pumps. I will also offer care guidelines for complications associated with breastfeeding such as cracked nipples, blocked ducts and mastitis, clues to whether your baby is getting enough milk, and how to manage supplemental feedings if necessary.

Benefits of Breastfeeding

There are many research-backed benefits of breastfeeding for you and your baby. To start with, breast milk perfectly meets the nutritional needs of your baby at each stage. It is readily available, which makes it easier for you to feed no matter where you are—no need to take along bottles, no quest to find warm, clean water, and no mixing or measuring! But in addition, breast milk lowers the risk factors of the following in babies:

- Ear infections
- Stomach viruses
- Food allergies
- Gas
- Diarrhea
- Respiratory infection
- Asthma
- Obesity
- Type 1 and 2 diabetes
- Childhood leukemia
- SIDS

Mothers who breastfeed receive benefits of their own, including:

- Less vaginal bleeding after delivery
- Easier loss of pregnancy weight
- Lower rate of type 2 diabetes
- Reduced risks of breast and ovarian cancer
- Improved bone density[34]

Rooming-In and Starting Out

. . . .

Immediately following delivery, your baby will most likely be quiet and alert—looking around, discovering her new environment, and getting to know her parents! As long as your and your baby's conditions are stable, you should start trying to breastfeed within the first hour or two. If you have a cesarean delivery and do not have enough energy to hold your baby, you can still have someone place your baby next to you to cuddle.

Relax and enjoy your first breastfeeding experience, whether your baby latches on right away or not. There is no reason to feel stress

---

34 Jan Riordan, *Breastfeeding and Human Lactation*, 3rd ed. (Sudbury, MA: Jones and Bartlett, 2005).

about anything, as keeping your baby at the breast, skin-to-skin, and giving her the opportunity to breastfeed is most important. Some babies are very eager to suckle and take milk, while others are satisfied with nuzzling at the breast and rooting at your nipple. Keep in mind that breastfeeding is a learning experience for your baby, and she may not be ready to latch on immediately after birth. Although you may feel drained emotionally and physically, you will probably be physically ready to breastfeed, and holding your newborn in your arms is the perfect reward for all your hard work and effort during the last nine months.

In order to maintain that important connection with your baby and set the stage for a successful breastfeeding experience, keep your baby in your room with you as much as possible during your first few days—whether you're in a hospital, birth center, or your own home. (This of course is providing everyone is healthy.) Some of the most reputable organizations, including the Academy of Breastfeeding Medicine, the American Academy of Pediatrics, and the American College of Obstetricians and Gynecologists recommend rooming-in, and recent research shows that limiting the amount of time a mother and baby stay together can negatively affect the breastfeeding experience. And because your baby should breastfeed approximately nine to twelve times in a twenty-four-hour period, rooming-in happens to be convenient! Your body responds better emotionally and physically to your baby's needs when close by, and research has found that moms who room in tend to:

- produce their milk sooner
- produce larger milk volumes
- breastfeed exclusively
- end up breastfeeding for a longer period

In addition, babies who room in tend to:
- have a lower chance of developing jaundice
- cry less often and be more easily consoled
- gain weight more steadily
- have better sleeping habits[35]

---

35   Cleveland Clinic, "Rooming-In: Rest Is Healing," my.clevelandclinic.org/health/articles/rooming-in-rest-is-healing.

baby care tip

If for health reasons you and your baby cannot room in together, be sure to have the nurse bring your baby to you for regular feedings at least every three hours. This will help ensure a long, successful breastfeeding experience with your baby once you are home.

Breast Physiology and Milk Production

There are three basic stages of breastfeeding: milk production, milk release, and milk transfer. All of these things need to happen in order to effectively nourish your baby. Milk production takes place in the alveoli, which are small sacs that form clusters called lobules (see Fig. 9-1). After the delivery of the placenta, your body will experience a rapid drop in progesterone and an increase in prolactin. These hormones work synergistically with others, including oxytocin, to establish and maintain lactation. When your baby begins feeding at the breast,

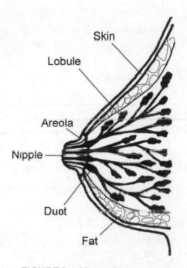

FIGURE 9-1: Human breast anatomy

the suckling stimulates your nerves and sends a signal to your brain, which then sends a message to the pituitary gland to release prolactin and oxytocin. Prolactin initiates the secretion of milk from the alveoli, and oxytocin causes milk to be released through the milk sinuses. This release is called the "letdown" or the "milk ejection reflex."

A delay in lactation can occur if these hormones are disrupted. Once lactation begins and the breast milk supply increases, the amount of milk produced depends on the amount of milk removed—that is why it is important to feed your newborn frequently. Each breast is a supply and demand system, operating independently from the other.

Changes in breast milk occur rapidly in the first few days after birth, and then slow down significantly. The three types of human milk are colostrum, transitional milk, and mature milk.

Colostrum—The first milk is thick, yellow, and high in protein, antibodies, vitamins, and minerals. Colostrum is usually produced during the first few days after birth, but some women may begin producing it a few days before.

Transitional milk—Thin and white in appearance, this milk contains high levels of fat, lactose, and water-soluble vitamins, and is higher in calories than colostrum. The content of this milk changes over the course of about ten to fifteen days, after which it is considered mature milk.

Mature milk—Composed of foremilk and hindmilk, mature milk fully comes in approximately two weeks after your baby's birth. Foremilk is high in protein and low in fat and calories, and, just as its name suggests, is the first of the mature milk to be secreted during each feeding. Hindmilk, which is produced toward the end of a feeding, is high in calories and fat. There is no one specific point in a feeding at which the milk changes from foremilk to hindmilk; it simply occurs when the fat that is stuck to the walls of the alveoli (where milk is made) begins to dislodge and secrete as the breast is emptied of its foremilk. It is important that babies receive a good balance of foremilk and hindmilk, and, as we'll see, feeding duration and milk supply help to ensure this.

baby care tip

Talk to your health-care provider about breastfeeding prior to delivery, and have your breasts and nipples examined. Enroll in a breastfeeding class if you can—taking these steps before your baby arrives will give you confidence in your ability to feed your baby. Yes, breastfeeding is natural and has been around forever, but it is not always automatic.

It is normal to feel worried about the size and shape of your breasts and nipples and concerned about whether or not they have the ability to provide adequate nourishment to your baby. Therefore, it is important for your provider to perform a prenatal breast assessment. The size and shape of your breasts usually do not affect lactation; in fact, most women's breasts are not symmetrical! However, there are some issues to be aware of. Here are some of the things your provider will be looking for and may discuss with you during the prenatal breast assessment:

Hypoplastic breasts—These breasts have underdeveloped milk glands. Breasts that lack normal fullness, are widely spaced, or appear tubular in shape may be associated with decreased milk supply.

Breast surgery—If you have had breast surgery, you may have some trouble producing enough milk. The movement and replacement of the nipple in surgery can damage nerves that are critical to the milk-making process. It will be important for you to check in with your health-care provider or lactation consultant in those early weeks if you are questioning your milk supply.

Inverted or flat nipples—Inverted or flat nipples may make it more difficult for your baby to latch on. A lactation consultant will be able to assess and assist you in latching your baby correctly.

baby care tip

It's easy to perform a self-assessment of your nipples. Just compress the areola between your forefinger and your thumb at the base of the nipple. A normal nipple will protrude or come out. If your nipple pulls in you could have inverted or flat nipples. Be sure to note if the surrounding tissue is firm or soft, as this may affect latch. Discuss your observations with your health-care provider.

Q. My nipples seem to be inverted. Will I still be able to breastfeed?

A. Inverted or flat nipples can make it more difficult for your baby to latch on, but this is not necessarily the case. If the tissue around the nipple is soft and pliable, the baby should be able to latch on just fine. Your baby will need to take in as much of the areola as possible, not just the nipple, to effectively extract the milk.

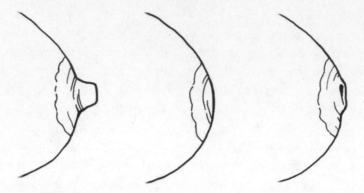

FIGURE 9-2: An everted nipple, a flat nipple, and an inverted nipple

Inverted nipples can often be pulled out by using a breast pump for a few minutes or by applying a cold cloth to help the nipple evert outward. This may be all it takes for your baby to get a good latch. You can also loosen the nipple tissue by placing your fingers one to two inches behind the nipple and pulling back into your chest. Breast shells have also become popular again. They are worn in the bra to draw out an otherwise flat nipple. They are very low cost, easy, and painless for moms with flatter nipples.

Remember, your breasts will change over time. The way your nipple looks on day two after birth could be very different from the way it looks on day seven. Also, if this is your second time breastfeeding you will probably have much less inversion this time around.

Q. My breasts are two different sizes. Is this normal?

A. Yes. In fact, most women's breasts are not symmetrical, and the number of milk-producing glands is not always equal between breasts. You may notice that one breast is producing a bit more milk than the other or that one breast is always a little fuller than the other. If this bothers you or is very noticeable, use a breast pump to stimulate the smaller breast for five minutes after each feed for a few days. Within two days you should notice a difference. If after this effort you still don't notice a change, that breast simply may not have as many milk-producing glands as the other breast—but no one will ever be able to tell!

Q. Why is colostrum referred to as "liquid gold"?

A. While colostrum's yellow-gold color contributes to its nickname, it's also called liquid gold because it's so valuable to your baby. Not only does it provide the nutrition your baby needs but it also provides protection by supplying your baby's first antibodies and immunities.

Colostrum can also be a huge help to mucusy babies. All babies swallow and breathe amniotic fluid while they are still in the womb. The transit through the birth canal squeezes a lot of this fluid out of the lungs, but some of it ends up being swallowed around the time of delivery, especially in the case of cesarean surgery. A belly or throat full of amniotic fluid will cause babies to sound mucusy and may make them gag when attempting to feed; it can even make a newborn feel full and uninterested in eating. Your colostrum loosens the mucus and helps clear it out of the body.

In addition, because colostrum is easily digested, it serves as a laxative and helps to clear a baby's digestive tract of any meconium she may have in her system.

Q. When will I begin to notice my milk supply increasing?

A. Within two to five days of birth, you will notice your breasts starting to feel more firm as your milk changes from colostrum to transitional milk. Your milk supply will increase depending on your baby's needs and by the amount of breastfeeding stimulation your body receives, which is why it is so important to keep your baby at the breast frequently throughout the day and night. Regular eating patterns and increased milk supply will also help him to gain weight.

If you had a cesarean section, you may notice that it takes another day or so for your milk supply to increase. This is normal. If your milk supply has not increased at all within seventy-two hours, though, talk to your baby's pediatrician and a lactation consultant for assistance. Remember, most babies lose up to 7 percent of their body weight in the first few days after birth!

Positioning and Latching at the Breast

· · · · · · · · · · · ·

Positioning your baby and getting him latched on to your breast and nipple correctly is one of the keys to successful breastfeeding. (This also happens to be the key to avoiding, or at least minimizing, nipple pain!) It is especially important during the early weeks of breastfeeding, when you and your baby are just getting the hang of it, to maintain proper positioning during feeds. If this is not your first breastfeeding experience, it is still very important to pay close attention to how you position your baby at the breast. Because your days-old baby still has very little muscle coordination and strength, he will need your help to achieve a good latch.

While you are still in the hospital, make sure an experienced nurse or lactation consultant observes you and your baby during a feeding session. If you are in a good breastfeeding position, you will be able to latch your baby on to the breast more effectively. Here are a few tips to ensuring a good position and latch:

- Find a comfortable, supportive place to sit.
- Put your feet up on a stool or add a few cushions under your feet to avoid bending toward your baby. Having your feet elevated will help you to achieve proper positioning.
- Whatever breastfeeding position you choose, bring your baby to your breast rather than your breast to your baby.
- Draw your baby toward you with his mouth wide open so that he receives enough milk, and to avoid a painful nipple-only latch.
- Align your baby's lower gum well below the base of the nipple on the areola, which allows him to compress the milk sinuses and draw out the milk.

Now, here are five traditional breastfeeding positions.

Cross-cradle hold—The cross-cradle hold is an ideal first position because it allows you to hold and control the position of your baby's head. Hold your baby along the opposite arm from the breast you are using. His body (tummy and chest) should be directly facing yours. In this position you can support your baby's neck and head with your hand, while your other hand can hold the breast and nipple in position to allow for easy latching. This will allow you to observe how your baby is latched on and, if necessary, make adjustments. Try to use a small blanket or rolled-up towel under the hand you are holding the baby's head with so your hand does not become tired. You can also use pillows on your lap to more easily keep your baby at the level of your breast.

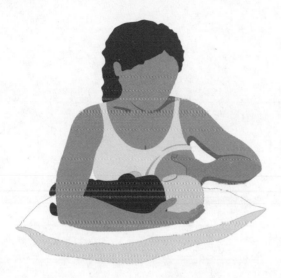

FIGURE 9-3: Cross-cradle breastfeeding hold

baby care tip

The cross-cradle hold is a great option in the first couple weeks after birth. Once your baby is properly latched, the hand that supports the breast can let go. This allows you a free hand in case you need to reposition the latch or wake up your baby by stimulating his feet and hands—or to finally sneak in a bite to eat!

Cradle hold—The cradle hold is a classic breastfeeding position and may be the most familiar to you. Place a few pillows on your lap and hold your baby's head in the crook of your elbow, supporting his back with your forearm. Tuck his lower hand under your arm and align his nose with your nipple.

Although this may seem like the most natural position, during the early days and weeks it is very difficult to control your baby's head using this hold. Once your baby is latching easily—and together you've mastered breastfeeding!—this will likely be the most comfortable and convenient position for you. I recommend the cradle hold when the baby is bigger and has more neck control, usually by the end of the first month. (Sometimes newborn infants can slide off. You will have more control and can keep your baby close in the cross-cradle hold.)

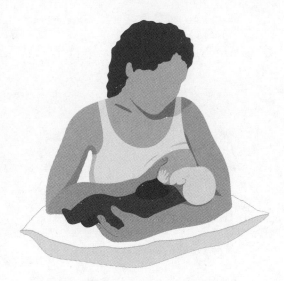

FIGURE 9-4: Cradle breastfeeding hold

Football hold—The football hold, as its name implies, positions your baby's body under your arm along your side, with his head at your breast and his feet toward your back as if you were holding a football. Again, as with all other breastfeeding positions, use plenty of pillows so that your baby is feeding at the level of your nipple and your arms don't become too tired, and make sure your baby is turned in toward you, his body facing yours. Your baby's head should be positioned just below the breast with his nose slightly above the nipple. Hold your free hand in a "C" position and compress the areola so that it matches the shape of your baby's mouth. When she opens her mouth wide, bring her to the breast and latch.

This position is often used during a baby's first few days if you cannot place him against your abdomen due to a C-section scar or pain in the area. Large-breasted women also find the football hold works well because the breast does not need to be supported for the baby to properly latch. Finally, if you are breastfeeding twins you can latch both babies onto the breast this way and feed them in tandem.

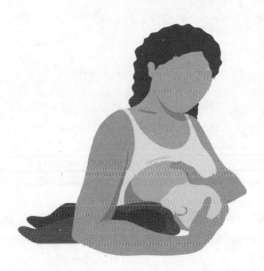

FIGURE 9-5: Football breastfeeding hold

Side-lying position—The side-lying position enables you to feed your baby in bed, which, as millions of moms can attest, is ideal for those midnight and early morning feedings! Lie down on your side and position your baby on her side as well, up close and facing you so that you're tummy to tummy. Use your hand to guide his mouth to your breast. Most women will use the lower breast, but if you have very large breasts you may be able to latch your baby to either the upper or the lower breast. You can support his back with your arm or place a rolled-up towel or blanket behind him to keep him in place. If your baby has a hard time latching on with this position, just wait a few weeks and try again. It will become much easier once your baby has more head control and can latch on without so much assistance.

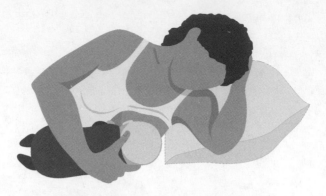

FIGURE 9-6: Side-lying breastfeeding position

Biological nursing—Also known as "laid-back breastfeeding," biological nursing promotes a baby's self-attaching reflexes. This is a hybrid, more relaxed breastfeeding position where mom gets into a comfortable semi-reclined position and the baby is placed on top, skin-to-skin. Then, gravity helps to activate the baby's primitive feeding reflexes, which can make a huge difference during the first few days of life when babies are at their most uncoordinated. The baby's body can be positioned in many different "laid-back" positions—there is no one "correct" angle or alignment with mom—making this a great option particularly after having a cesarean birth.

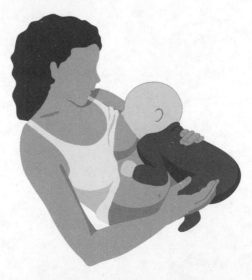

FIGURE 9-7: Laid-back breastfeeding position

baby care tip

When using the laid-back breastfeeding position, it's best for mom to find the ideal positioning that works for her. More often than not, this happens through trial and error (and patience!). If you're interested in trying this approach, avoid straining to mimic specific positions and, instead, spend significant time with baby near or lying on your breast, which can ultimately help both of you determine which position works best.

In order to get off to a good start, breastfeed in the position where your baby has the best latch and you are the most comfortable. When your baby is positioned properly at the breast, you may feel a bit of pain during latch-on but little to no pain when he is feeding. If you do feel ongoing pain, engage the help of a nurse or lactation consultant. Get really good at one position during the first few days and weeks instead of trying to learn every breastfeeding position you've read about. (In other words, if the very first position you try works well, stick to it! If it doesn't work, change positions until you find one that does!) You may also find that you use a different hold for each breast. As you and your baby get more comfortable and feel more at ease with breastfeeding, different positions will become natural to you. Believe it or not, within a few weeks you will feel comfortable and confident with breastfeeding, making it an experience of bonding and well-being for both of you.

baby care tip

Break the latch gently! When your baby is sucking with force but doesn't have the right latch, or you just want to take him off the breast, simply edge your pinky finger slowly in between the corner of your baby's mouth and your nipple. This will break the suction of the latch and avoid painful irritation and damage to your nipple.

Feeding Frequency and Duration

. . . .

Your baby should breastfeed approximately nine to twelve times in a twenty-four-hour period. Your newborn may not seem to be interested in eating on his very first day, but you will still be expected to attempt feedings at a minimum of every three hours even if that means waking your baby up. I know that seems unkind to everyone involved, but it's not! Parents commonly feel that if their newborn is sleeping quietly, he must not be hungry. This is not the case with a newborn, at least for the first few weeks and maybe even longer. In fact, dehydrated babies are more sleepy and harder to wake. You will be much more successful in feeding him if you wake him up and get him eager to feed with a wide mouth. So-called demand feeding, in which you respond to your baby's hunger cues, should not happen until your baby begins regularly waking on his own for feedings.

Q. How often should I breastfeed my newborn during the first twenty-four hours?

A. The more time spent at the breast, the better, as it helps both you and your baby to get used to breastfeeding. Try to feed roughly every three hours, for a total of about eight sessions during the first twenty-four hours. (Your baby will take approximately 7.5 to 10 milliliters per feeding during this time.) If you can, attempt to breastfeed your baby within the first hour or so after birth. Remember, some babies are ready to feed and will latch on to the breast with ease, and others for whatever reason take a bit longer—but it's crucial that you continue to try. One of the best ways to get your baby interested in breastfeeding is to give him as much skin-to-skin contact as possible.

baby care tip

Your hospital stay will be short, so learn as much as you can from the experts. In addition to getting guidance about your breastfeeding position and your baby's latch, ask them to go over common newborn feeding issues with you and, of course, any specific questions you may have.

Q. What kind of feeding schedule should I follow once I get home from the hospital?

A. For at least the first couple of weeks, feed your newborn baby every one to three hours throughout the day and night—about nine to twelve times a day. (It's OK to have one long stretch of about four hours during the night.) Babies tend to be very sleepy, especially during daytime hours, so be sure to wake your baby up for feedings. The more she feeds during the day, the less hungry she will be at night.

You can keep your baby at the breast for up to thirty minutes if she is sucking vigorously, and then you can offer the other breast. If she chooses to take only one breast at a feeding, make sure you begin the next feeding session with the other breast. Remember that every baby is different and some feed effectively in a shorter time. Leave the baby on the first breast until she comes off on her own.

baby care tip

Keep track! Breastfeeding during your first week or so home will be exhausting and it may be difficult to remember which breast you offered your baby last. It can be helpful to keep a pad of paper and a pen next to your nursing chair so you can record the time and side you last fed with. This will help to ensure timely feedings (and healthy weight gain for your baby!) and avoid engorgement.

Q. Should I change my baby's diaper before or after I breastfeed him?

A. During the early weeks it's a good idea to have your baby wide awake and eager to eat when you start your breastfeeding session. Changing a diaper will help you to accomplish that. Most babies do not like to be moved around much, so unswaddle your baby, rub his tummy, move his arms and legs a bit, and then change the diaper. Of course, if your baby dirties a diaper while you're feeding it is generally a good idea to go ahead and change him—keeping him in a soiled (poopy) diaper will not be comfortable for him and can lead to diaper rash.

Q. My friend told me that she breastfed her baby for ten minutes per breast during a feeding and suggested I do the same. How long should I keep my baby on a breast before switching sides?

A. This advice is not correct, and may result in a gassy and fussy baby. Breast milk changes throughout the feeding session. During the first part of the feed, the breast milk (foremilk) contains more water. This helps to quench the baby's thirst and begin to fill her stomach. As the feeding continues, the breast milk changes to hindmilk, which contains more fat. This fat is important to help the baby digest the breast milk, and it also makes the baby feel full at the end of a feeding—it's often compared to having a piece of rich cheesecake after dinner!

A good way to tell whether your baby is getting enough hindmilk is through stool color and consistency—if her stools are consistently very green and mucusy, she may not be. To ensure that your baby does receive a good balance of foremilk and hindmilk, feed her on one side until the breast is completely drained and feels soft (up to thirty minutes). If your baby is satisfied and sleeping he has probably had enough, but if not, continue feeding on the other breast. (It is fine if your baby only feeds for a few minutes on the second breast.) Alternate the starting breast with each feed.

Q. My baby is three weeks old and gaining weight steadily. Do I still have to wake him every few hours to feed?

A. If your baby is three weeks old, breastfeeding well, and steadily gaining weight, it's all right to let him sleep longer between feedings, and feed on demand. Your baby will eventually determine the frequency and duration of breastfeeding sessions. It is better for you and your baby to have most of his nutritional needs met during the day so you are not playing catch-up at night with a hungry baby. You should still be breastfeeding about every three hours and let him have his long stretches of sleep at night instead of the day. Sometimes babies will have growth spurts though—commonly seen at two weeks and six weeks. During this time, your baby may be demanding more food and breastfeeding more often.

Feeding Schedules

Ultimately you need to come up with a lifestyle, routine, or schedule that works for you and for your baby. While it is not recommended to have a baby of less than three weeks on a schedule because of her unpredictable eating needs and small stomach capacity, by the end of the second or third week your baby may have a growth spurt and you may see an increase in appetite. After this, your baby will become more active and stay awake a bit longer. Her stomach capacity will increase and you'll begin to notice feeding patterns becoming more predictable. If you want to begin a flexible feeding schedule, this is the time to do it. In my experience, babies who adapt to a feeding schedule tend to have a more regular sleeping pattern as well.

Keep in mind that every new mom is different, just as every baby is different. Some moms are not interested in the clock and are comfortable feeding on demand. Other moms like to have some routine in their daily activities. We will discuss newborn routines and scheduling later in the book, with sample schedules that you can try to follow during your baby's first, second, and third month. Try to have a relaxed attitude and don't overthink things. Remember that even if you begin to initiate a flexible daily feeding schedule, you will have some days when, for whatever reason, you just can't stick to it. This is to be expected, not just in the early weeks but also as your baby grows. Just when you think things are running smoothly, your baby will want to change things up and it may take a few days to get back on track—if a completely new track has not been set, that is!

Q. My baby is so sleepy during the day that it can be difficult to keep him awake throughout a feeding. But at ten o'clock at night, when I'm ready to go to sleep, my baby wakes up and wants to nurse all the time. Is there anything I can do to curb this?

A. Many newborns take one long, restful stretch of sleep of about four to five hours in a twenty-four-hour period. Unfortunately, for the first few weeks most prefer to take this long nap in the daytime instead of at night—that is, if you let them! This is opposite of your own sleep needs and can make for very tired parents, which makes it in your best interest to try to develop similar sleep cycles.

There are some things you can do to help your baby sleep more during the nighttime hours. Feed and wake your baby more often during the day, as it will help to change his internal clock. He will gradually begin to be more awake during the day and sleep for longer stretches at night. Studies show that newborns develop their own circadian rhythms a few weeks after birth. Exposure to light helps influence your baby's sleeping patterns just as it influences yours. Keep your shades open during the day to let the light in; don't keep your home dark because you want your baby to nap. Conversely, try to limit the use of bright lights when you're feeding during the night. A nightlight can help you to see while also keeping the room dim.

baby care tip

Don't try to keep the house quiet or dark during the day for your baby to nap. While your baby is sleeping, he'll still be aware of daytime noises such as talking, music, and telephones ringing. At night, go ahead and quiet things down; the lights can be dimmed and activities slowed. This is how your baby will begin to change his internal clock.

Waking Techniques

I've already covered the subject of waking your newborn to eat regularly, but it warrants reiteration. The fact is, your baby needs to eat every one to three hours and it's your job as parents to feed him, asleep or not. I agree that sometimes it is very difficult to wake a sleepy baby, especially during the first twenty-four hours after birth. However, the longer he goes without food, the less energy he will have and the sleepier he will be. This can be a difficult cycle to break.

baby care tip

Here are a few ways to wake your baby, whether for breastfeeding purposes or for the sake of getting him on a good sleep/wake cycle— the two go hand in hand!

- Unwrap or unswaddle him from his blankets
- Undress him down to his diaper
- Change the diaper, even if it is dry

- Sit your baby up on your lap, holding him under his chin, and gently rub his back
- Stroke his face with a cool washcloth
- Let him suck on your finger to get him ready to latch
- Change his position away from the comfort of your body—place him on a bed, changing table, or bassinet (anywhere safe, but not on your warm skin)
- Rub his arms and legs and massage his feet
- Be persistent

Birth Weight Loss and Supplementation

Your baby will likely lose several ounces during the first few days after delivery—this is completely normal. The loss should turn around once your milk supply begins to increase, usually between the third and sixth day postpartum. If you had a cesarean delivery, you may not feel breast fullness until the fifth or sixth day after delivery. If, for some reason, it seems your baby is not taking in any food, you may have to supplement with formula.

Sometimes babies have a difficult time taking in enough breast milk due to a condition called ankyloglossia, in which tongue movement is restricted as a result of an abnormally short or tight frenulum (the skin that attaches the tongue to bottom of the mouth). Lactation consultants can usually pick up on this condition and will discuss your options with you along with your care provider. There is a procedure that can be done to release the tongue called a frenotomy; however, a review of breastfeeding outcomes by the AAP published in the journal *Pediatrics* in 2015 concluded that there is little evidence supporting its efficacy.[36] Furthermore, it is possible for the frenulum to stretch on its own as your baby continues feeding throughout his first weeks.

---

36   D. O. Francis, S. Krishnaswami, and M. McPheeters, "Treatment of Ankyloglossia and Breastfeeding Outcomes: A Systematic Review," *Pediatrics* 135, no. 6 (June 2015). pediatrics.aappublications.org/content/early/2015/04/28/peds.2015-0658.

Q. How do I know that my baby is getting enough to eat?

A. Not knowing how much milk is being consumed during a feeding is probably the biggest concern that new parents have about their newborns—if only breasts had ounce markers as bottles do! I know the uncertainty can be unnerving at times. Just try to relax and make sure to feed your baby at least once every three hours. Your baby will likely get enough milk if he is nursing between fifteen and forty-five minutes at each feeding and seems content when he is finished. When your breasts begin to fill you may hear your baby swallow, and when he gets milk he will take long, rhythmic sucks. You may notice that your baby is in a pattern of taking five to ten continuous sucks followed by a brief pause; this is the swallow.

Your breast will be much softer and lighter after the baby has fed—this is one sign that milk has been transferred to your baby. Another way to monitor consumption is to check your baby's diaper. During the first few days, your baby should have regular bowel movements but urinate rather infrequently. After approximately five days, his stool should begin to change to a yellow color and wet diapers should start to increase. These are all clear signs that the baby is getting enough food. Of course, you should follow up with your baby's pediatrician for a routine newborn appointment to have your baby weighed after you're discharged from the hospital, typically within a day or two.

baby care tip

Here is the normal output for breastfeeding infants in a twenty-four-hour period.

Birth to four days old—Two to five stool diapers, and one more wet diaper than the number of days old (e.g., three days old = four wet diapers)

Five days and older—One or more stool diaper (stool will change from dark meconium to a mustard color in the first week), and six or more wet diapers

Q. My baby has lost weight: He was eight pounds five ounces at birth, and now on day two he's down to eight pounds. Is this normal? When will he start to gain weight?

A. Yes, this is absolutely normal for infants and nothing to worry about. Why? One common theory is that babies are born with a little extra weight to help them deal with the stress caused by labor and birth, and to help them through those first few days of life when their mother's milk supply is low. The use of IV fluids in labor may also increase the baby's fluid intake, and this contributes to a higher weight immediately after birth. After the fifth day of life a baby should gain between a half and a full ounce per day. Your baby's pediatrician will be monitoring his weight at your newborn visits. Many babies regain their birth weight by two weeks of age.

Q. My baby has lost 10 percent of his birth weight and the pediatrician is recommending that I supplement my feedings with formula. I am upset—did I do something wrong?

A. No, you had nothing to do with this weight loss. A baby can lose too much weight if the mother's milk doesn't come in by the third or fourth day, if nursing is infrequent, or if he is not nursing effectively. Your baby's pediatrician may recommend giving the baby a supplement of formula or expressed breast milk, if available. Supplementing with formula, if medically necessary, should not interfere with successful breastfeeding. There are several feeding methods that do not involve a bottle, if nipple confusion is a concern.

When a baby loses 10 percent of his weight he may become more tired than usual, and this will interfere with his ability to nurse long enough to gain his weight back. This can create a dangerous cycle, so talk to your pediatrician about how much supplementation is necessary and for how long. Sometimes it is just for twenty-four hours—enough time for your milk supply to increase. In addition to supplementation, make sure that you have a skilled nurse or lactation consultant observe you and your baby breastfeeding. A baby who is not latched properly may look like he is feeding when in fact not much milk is being transferred. You can also ask about the possibility of using a breast pump to help increase your milk supply.

Q. My baby breastfed fine for the first two days, but this morning she is fussy and irritable and I cannot get her to latch. Last night I sent her to the nursery and asked the nurses to feed her a bottle so I could sleep. Why is she now so fussy?

A. There are a few reasons why your baby could be having a hard time breastfeeding. The fact that she spent some time in the nursery is not a problem, but having a bottle of formula can affect how a baby reacts at the breast.

To get milk from the breast, a baby needs to latch correctly and coordinate her tongue and jaw movement to suck in a way that is unique to breastfeeding. When your baby takes a bottle she does not have to latch properly, and thanks to gravity the formula will flow into her mouth immediately, satisfying her in seconds. Compare this to breastfeeding, where your baby has to suck properly for a minute or two before she gets the milk flowing. The problem this morning is that your baby is expecting milk from your breast the same way she got it from the bottle. This can be very frustrating for both of you. Be patient and continue trying to latch your baby—she will go back to the breast, but you may need to work a bit harder to get her to feed effectively there.

Make sure to calm your baby down before trying to breastfeed her. Place her on your chest and hold her skin-to-skin. Insert your finger in her mouth and let her suck on it until she relaxes, and then try to latch. Express some drops of colostrum onto her lips while she is trying to latch. If these techniques don't work, ask your health-care provider, nurse, or lactation consultant to help you. Your baby will go back onto the breast—she just needs some patient guidance.

Alternatives to the Bottle

If you are committed to breastfeeding and want to get off to a good start, do not introduce either a bottle or formula unless they are medically indicated and recommended by your baby's pediatrician. If your pediatrician does recommend supplementation and your breast milk supply is not yet sufficient, there are ways to feed your baby without the use of a bottle. Finger feeding, cup feeding, and supplemental nursing systems (SNS) work very well and can be an effective way to feed your baby without interfering with breastfeeding. You can ask the hospital staff to teach you how to cup- or finger feed your baby. When choosing a feeding method, it's always best to talk to an experienced health-care provider or lactation consultant.

Cup feeding—This technique involves placing the rim of a small medicine cup on the baby's lower lip and tipping the cup slightly so that the baby can slowly sip or lap the milk or formula. This type of feeding method has been gaining popularity in many hospitals as an alternative to bottles. Many countries around the world routinely use this type of feeding method and the World Health Organization advocates it when necessary. Recent studies have also proven cup feeding to be safe and effective in preterm infants. Your health care provider will show you how to safely use this alternative feeding method.

Finger feeding—This method involves placing a thin plastic tube on the parent's finger, sometimes attached with a small piece of tape to keep it in place. The tube is connected to a device that has a small amount of formula or expressed breast milk. As the baby sucks on the finger, he receives milk or formula. The finger has a more natural feel than a rubber nipple, and the flow of milk can be made to mimic the breastfeeding flow.

Supplemental nursing system (SNS)—This device consists of a small container for the supplement and a long, thin tube that you slide into the baby's mouth while he is latched at the breast. Some hospitals may use a syringe and attach a tube to make the feeding device. The baby will get your milk and the supplementation at the same time. As with the other feeding methods, an experienced health-care provider or lactation consultant should teach you how to do this.

Milk Expression and Storage

At some point you might choose to express, or pump, your breast milk for a variety of reasons, including:
- Your baby is premature
- Your baby is unable to breastfeed
- You are ill and unable to breastfeed

- You are returning to work
- You want a supply of milk for times when you are away
- You want to increase your milk supply
- You want to relieve engorgement

Q. Should I buy a breast pump before I have my baby?

A. It may be a good idea to wait until after your baby is born to purchase a breast pump. If your health-care provider or lactation nurse recommends pumping your breasts while you are in the hospital, the staff will set you up with a pump and the necessary equipment. If your health-care provider recommends that you continue using a breast pump after your discharge, check with your insurance company to see if they provide some type of reimbursement. If not, you can usually purchase or rent a breast pump fairly quickly and easily. Most hospitals either have rental programs or work with medical supply companies that rent and sell breast pumps. Many retailers and baby stores also carry a wide selection of breast pumps—even quiet, hands-free ones that are especially great for pumping at work! Ask your hospital nurse or lactation consultant for recommendations.

Breast Pumps

Manual breast pump—Light, portable, and affordable, manual breast pumps are great for on-the-go use, or if you're only planning on pumping occasionally when you'll be away from baby for short periods of time. It can also be helpful when you're particularly full and need to release a bit of breast milk before a feeding to help baby get an easier latch. The handheld pump comes with a breast shield (flange), bottle with lid and stand, a valve, and a couple membranes.

Pros: Low-cost, quiet, convenient
Cons: Slow, more physical work, pumps one breast at a time

Single electric breast pump—Single electric breast pumps cost more than manual pumps—you can find them for around $100—but they can be well worth the investment, as they require less work on your end, help produce more breast milk in less time, and are still fairly compact. They typically have a few different settings of expression speed so you can use what's comfortable for you. Most can be electric or battery operated, depending on where you are.

Pros: Relatively low cost, portable, quick production

Cons: Loud, pumps one breast at a time

Double electric breast pump—Double electric breast pumps are an asset to moms who are having a little trouble breastfeeding or are planning to return to work while breastfeeding. Like the single electric breast pump, this pump has several expression settings, but since it pumps from two breasts at the same time, it can produce much more breast milk. They typically come with a carrying case, tubing, bottles, two shields, valves, and membranes.

Pros: Quick production, minimal effort

Cons: Can be expensive, loud, cumbersome

Hands-free double electric pump—Hands-free electric pumps are great for moms who need to pump outside of the home frequently. Like other electric models, they are quick to produce and have various expression settings to suit mom's comfort level. The most modern models are discrete—pumping quietly *under* your clothes—providing a more pleasant experience for moms.

Pros: Discrete, quick production

Cons: Can be expensive

baby care tip

Technically any double pump can be a hands-free pump. It just means you have to purchase a hands-free bra.

Hospital-grade pump—These pumps are generally faster and more powerful, which is why hospitals use these pumps for multiple mothers while they are in the hospital. Most mothers choose not to purchase a hospital-grade pump, as they are readily available for rental. Check your insurance policy to see whether or not you qualify to rent a pump.

Pros: Fast, powerful, and efficient, most likely pumping more per session than any hand pump or single-use pump.

Cons: Expensive to purchase unless your insurance qualifies you for rental, loud, not portable, cumbersome and difficult to assemble

Smart pumps—These breast pumps make every other pump look outdated by comparison. Instead of requiring assembly of an apparatus with many parts to connect and disconnect, the new smart pumps consist of an integrated system without cords, wires, or tubes to worry about. It is unclear if these smart pumps will initially be as effective as their older counterparts, but these new innovations will certainly simplify the breast-pumping experience.

Q. I would like to start pumping so I can begin to store extra milk in case I need to be away from my baby for a while. What is the best way to go about this?

A. Many mothers find it convenient to have a supply of breast milk stored for future use. Expressing milk can be done by hand or with the use of a manual or electric breast pump. Whatever method you choose, make sure you wash your hands well with soap and water before starting and make sure your collection containers are clean. Read the instruction book that comes with your pump before you get started.

Try waiting until breastfeeding is going well before introducing a bottle of expressed milk to your baby. It usually takes a few weeks for mothers and babies to get really good at breastfeeding. Although sucking is a newborn reflex, the mechanics of effectively latching need to be learned, and, as we have seen, introducing a bottle too early can get in the way of that process.

When you first begin to pump you will not express much extra milk, as your body is making just enough to feed your baby. When you begin pumping, you are essentially placing an order, and it takes several days for your body to make more milk in response. Begin pumping once or twice a day right after you finish breastfeeding your baby. Morning is a good time to start pumping because your milk supply tends to be greatest at that time. Pump each breast for approximately ten to fifteen minutes, whether you are pumping both or just one breast. You may not see much milk initially, but you are sending a signal to the brain to increase your milk supply. You can pump again in the early afternoon and before you go to bed. Be consistent and pump at approximately the same time every day. Within a few days you will notice that your milk supply is increasing, and you will be able to pump extra milk that you can store for later use. Remember, though, that breast milk production is a result of supply and demand. If you feel that your supply has increased too much, cut down on the number of times you use your breast pump.

If you are preparing to return to work, begin pumping three to four weeks in advance. It takes some time for your body to begin producing enough breast milk for you to feed your baby and have enough left over for storage. You will also want to introduce bottles of expressed breast milk between weeks three and six so that your baby gets accustomed to this type of feeding. One bottle a day should be all that is needed to accomplish this.

baby care tip

Freshly expressed breast milk can be safely stored for hours, days, or months depending on the conditions.

Room temperature: four to six hours at 66–78°F (19–26°C)

Cooler with three ice or gel packs: twenty-four hours at 59°F (15°C)

Refrigerator: three to eight days at 39°F (1°C)

Freezer: six to twelve months at 0–4°F (–18 to –20°C)

Thawed after freezing: Use within twenty-four hours[37]

Q. I've just started pumping and my nipples are very sore. What can I do?

A. You may experience some nipple tenderness when you first begin pumping. This usually goes away within a few days. There are some things that you can do to help prevent soreness:

- Massage your breasts for a few minutes before you pump to help get the milk flowing.
- Apply a warm compress or take a warm shower to soften the breasts.
- Make sure the flanges fit properly and are not irritating the area between the nipple and the areola.
- Make sure the setting on the pump is not too high.

---

37   Medela, "Collection and Storage of Breast Milk," medelabreastfeedingus.com/tips-and-solutions/11/breastmilk-collection-and-storage.

- Apply some breast milk to nipples after each pumping session and let them air dry.
- Do not keep wet nursing pads next to your nipples.

Common Breastfeeding Concerns

I can't reiterate enough how many perfectly normal little hiccups you may run into while learning how to breastfeed your baby. Here are a few common breastfeeding issues that I've seen time and time again—and some solutions to help get through them.

Sore Nipples

Nipple soreness and discomfort during the first few days is very discouraging and can put a damper on the joys of breastfeeding. Newborns tend to have a very strong suck during those first few days in order to draw the colostrum, so slight tenderness is normal. If your baby is latched correctly, your soreness will most likely go away when the milk supply increases, around day seven to ten, because the baby will not have to suck as strongly to get milk. By days three and four your nipples will start to feel more comfortable during each feeding. If you continue to have sore nipples, however, here are a few recommendations.

- Massage your breasts to express a few drops of colostrum or breast milk so that they coat your nipple. Human milk has antibacterial properties that can help to heal an inflamed nipple.
- Make sure your baby is properly positioned at the breast. If using the cross or cradle holds, make sure your baby completely faces you and you are holding him close. Drawing your baby close helps him to get more of the areola into his mouth.
- Make sure you bring your baby to the breast with his mouth wide open and centered over the areola when latching. If you feel a pinch, use your finger to gently pull down on his chin and roll out the lower lip.

- Feed your baby frequently so he is not overly hungry. If he is very hungry, he may be so frantic that he begins to pull at the nipple.
- If you can, avoid pacifiers and artificial bottle nipples for at least a few weeks. They may contribute to your baby incorrectly sucking at the breast.
- Apply breast milk to your nipples following each feeding and let them air dry. Avoid creams and lotions unless medically indicated.
- If your nipples are not healing, contact your health-care provider or a lactation consultant so they can observe one of your breastfeeding sessions.

baby care tip

If your breasts don't typically leak throughout the day, you can save money on disposable breast pads—and time spent washing reusable cotton ones—by only using one (don't worry; because these tend to be thin, this won't make you look lopsided). When you're feeding on the right side, place the breast pad on your left breast to absorb the letdown milk. The next time you feed, simply switch the pad to the other side. Wearing a pad can also help you keep track of which side your baby last fed on!

Engorgement

Engorgement is like rush hour traffic at your breasts. This swelling, which usually happens only once, is caused not only by the accumulation of milk but also by an increased blood flow to the breasts. Your breasts will start to become heavy and full anywhere from two to six days postpartum. Not all women experience the same degree of swelling—some women have breasts that feel hard as rocks and others just notice a supple fullness. The period of marked engorgement typically lasts one or two days, but it can take up to two weeks to recede completely. Feeding your baby often without limiting time at the breast, and breastfeeding exclusively without offering supplements, can help to prevent severe engorgement. You may experience more swelling and edema (excess accumulation of fluid in your body tissue) if you received excessive intravenous fluids during your labor.

TREATMENTS FOR ENGORGEMENT

- **Heat before the feeding**—Using heat prior to feeding helps to soften the tissue and helps the milk let down. Taking a warm shower and using warm compresses on the breasts works well.

- **Cold after the feeding**—Use cold compresses on your breasts, such as frozen vegetable bags or ice packs, after breastfeeding. The cold will help reduce the swelling in your breasts, which should provide you with some relief.

- **Breast massage and milk expression**—Massage your breasts and express milk to relieve some pressure.

- **Pumping**—Use a manual or electric breast pump for a few minutes to help soften the breasts. But do not overuse the breast pump because it may increase your milk supply too much.

- **Cabbage leaves**—Apply cabbage leaves to your breasts between feedings. No one knows exactly why this works but it is a remedy that has been used for years. Cool the cabbage in the refrigerator and then cut in half. Remove the leaves and place around the breast (they will actually fit nicely). Keep them on for up to thirty minutes. When you feel the milk start to leak, put your baby to the breast.

- **Areolar compression**—Reduce edema around the nipple so baby can latch. Ask your health-care provider to show you this technique.

- **Nurse frequently during this time**—Try to breastfeed ten to twelve times in a twenty-four-hour period. Do not go longer than three hours between feedings—not even during the night.

- **Try to breastfeed your baby in a different position**—If you've been using the cross-cradle position for breastfeeding, try the football hold. This may promote more milk removal.

Blisters

A blister, which is a collection of clear fluid under the skin, can form on the nipple or areola of the breast in response to the friction of the baby's tongue on the skin. They are usually not painful or worrisome, and there is no treatment—just leave them alone, as they usually heal eventually.

A milk blister is not the same as a blister caused by friction. Sometimes a milk blister shows up as a painful white or yellow dot on the nipple or areola, in which case it is called a blocked nipple pore or a bleb. These types of blisters can be persistent and painful during feeding sessions. They form when milk within the duct has been sealed over by the epidermis, causing the white or yellow spot. Sometimes an oversupply of milk may cause these blisters; at other times, problems with the latch or suck can contribute. The bleb may last for several days or weeks and then spontaneously heal.

To treat one, apply a warm compress to the blister prior to breast-feeding—the combination of heat and breastfeeding should cause the skin to expand, and the blister to eventually open. You may need to contact your health-care provider if the blister does not go away.

Blocked Ducts

Blocked (or plugged) ducts are red, tender, pea-sized areas under the skin of the breast, usually caused by skipped or delayed feedings. They can also result from an overabundant milk supply, an underwire bra that puts too much pressure over a duct, or nursing your baby in a poor position. Apply warm compresses to the affected area and breast-feed frequently. Gently massaging the affected area while nursing or taking a warm shower may help relieve some pressure as well.

baby care tip

Position your baby so that his chin is facing the blocked duct. This allows for more milk removal in the affected area. You may need to be somewhat creative in finding a comfortable position for both you and the baby.

Mastitis

If a blocked duct persists, it could become inflamed and turn into a breast infection. If you begin to develop a red area on your breast and/or flulike symptoms that include a fever, headache, weakness, chills, and achy muscles, contact your health-care provider right away. A prescribed antibiotic will usually make you feel better within forty-eight hours. Yes, you should still breastfeed; in fact, nursing frequently will help to relieve your discomfort. Just as with a blocked duct, treatment involves warm compresses to the affected area, plenty of rest, lots of fluids, and antibiotic therapy.

Yeast Infection

Yeast infections are also known as thrush and candidiasis. Yeast can be found in the birth canal, and as a result, babies can become infected during a vaginal delivery. Signs of a yeast infection usually appear a few weeks after the birth. On the baby you will notice small white patches in the mouth and possibly a bright red rash on his bottom. You, in turn, can become infected while breastfeeding, in which case you will notice small red or white patches on the breast. You may also experience a shooting pain during the feeding. Sometimes this is the only symptom.

Both you and your baby will need to be treated to prevent reinfection. Anti-yeast medication will be prescribed by your provider, usually an ointment for your breasts and a liquid for the baby. Your provider will show you how to apply the liquid in and around the baby's mouth. If your baby has a rash, you may be instructed to use the ointment on the baby's bottom as well.

Breastfeeding a Preterm Baby

Most parents don't expect to give birth to a premature baby. A baby delivered prior to 37 weeks is considered premature. Babies who are delivered between three and six weeks early are called late preterm babies. These babies do not eat as much as full-term babies and may need to be fed more often. They may also have some trouble coordinating sucking and swallowing. Babies born at less than 37 weeks are also sleepier and have less energy than full-term babies.

Hospital staff are knowledgeable in this area and will assist you in choosing the best feeding method for your baby. A baby should have at least 32 to 33 weeks' gestation before breastfeeding can begin, so prior to this time your baby may be fed with a feeding tube of formula or expressed breast milk. Your baby's health-care team will encourage breastfeeding because breast milk is especially important to your preterm baby. If you deliver prematurely, your milk will be slightly different than if you carry to term. "Premature milk" is especially beneficial for your baby and provides extra protection against some of the problems that premature babies may develop.

You will need to express milk with an electric pump within twenty-four hours of the birth to stimulate milk production. Don't worry about buying a breast pump yet, as the hospital will have one for you to use. Pump your breasts every three hours for approximately fifteen minutes and your breasts will start to produce milk.

Checking in with Dad (or Partner)

Dads and partners: If your baby is breastfed, you may feel a little helpless at first. Although you want to help, it may seem like there's not a lot you can do. But while you won't be able to take part in feedings directly, as many fathers of formula-fed babies can, here are a few ways to get involved right from the start.

- Help make Mom comfortable by setting up pillows around her, and put a glass of water next to her to help keep her hydrated.
- Hold and talk to your baby while Mom settles in.
- Hand your baby to Mom for the feeding and provide any positioning assistance she might need.
- Burp your baby for Mom. This is especially useful if Mom had a cesarean birth.
- If your baby is sleepy and not feeding for long enough, massage and gently compress your partner's breasts to help the milk flow. Once the baby starts getting a steady flow of milk, he will probably become more interested in feeding.
- Especially important in the first week or so: keep track of the time and duration of each feed as well as on which breast the last feeding took place. This will help ensure that your baby gets enough to eat, and prevent engorgement and discomfort for Mom.

Although I always discuss the benefits of exclusively breastfeeding with new parents, I know that some will ultimately have to take another path that works best for them—and that's OK. There are some mothers who, for whatever reason, cannot or choose not to breastfeed. For some women breastfeeding does not fit into their lifestyle or parenting philosophy, while others simply can't breastfeed because of medical conditions or because they take medications. Other women decide to breastfeed and supplement their breast milk with formula. But no matter the method you choose, you will bond with your baby during feedings. No one loves your baby more than you, his parents, do, and your feeding decision is yours and yours alone to make. Your health-care providers and others around you should support the decisions you make. Choosing not to breastfeed or not to exclusively breastfeed does not make you a bad mother, and you should not feel guilty or somehow condemned about your choices. You know what is best for your baby and that will make you a terrific parent.

PART IV

The Fourth Trimester

· 10 ·

Your Baby's First Month: A Time for Learning

Coming home with your baby will be one of the most exciting moments in your new life as a parent. This will be a magical stage when you will begin the important bonding process with your infant. Understand that your baby has a unique personality and temperament and it will take some time for you to get to know each other. It is normal to feel overwhelmed with both joy and the new sense of responsibility. This chapter is designed to guide you through your first month at home together, providing information you'll need to be able to relax and enjoy your baby. We'll cover feeding, soothing, sleeping, development, milestones, what's going on with you, and checking in with Dad/Partner. It also includes suggested daily routines for you to follow to help make your days and nights manageable.

Although bringing home your new baby is an exciting moment for your new family, you may feel some fear about leaving the secure hospital environment, where professionals were available 24/7 to answer any questions and concerns you had about your newborn. You may even feel unprepared to care for your baby. Rest assured that this feeling is entirely normal, and you and your baby will do just fine. An inner wisdom will take over (both moms and dads have this) and you *will* know how to care for your baby.

First Days at Home

· · · · · · · · · · · · ·

Here are some recommended housekeeping measures to help you get settled comfortably: When you arrive home, ask your partner to help you set up a "nest." This is where you will do a lot of your daytime feeding and will sit and rest with your baby while you're awake. Make sure it's a comfortable spot, such as a couch or a rocker or glider. Some helpful things to have nearby are snacks, a water bottle, your cell phone, and the house phone if you have one, although, of course, it's perfectly acceptable to turn off your phones if you want some well-earned peace and quiet! When at home, dress in comfortable clothes—even pajamas—for the first few days. You will have a lot of recovering to do.

Q. People are so excited to see the baby, but all they want to do is hold her. This makes me feel stressed—what can I do?

A. It is best for a newborn to stay close to her parents as much as possible during those first few weeks—this provides her with a stable foundation based on bonding, comfort, and familiarity. It's not a problem to let *healthy* family members or a few close friends hold your newborn for a short time but I recommend keeping the constant passing around to a minimum. In addition to possible germ exposure, the movement may be too stimulating for your days-old baby. At around one to two months old you won't need to be so careful.

It is perfectly fine to set limits on both the number of visitors and rules about who holds your baby and when. If you cannot limit your visitors or you feel uncomfortable telling visitors how you feel, put your sleeping baby in a bassinet or crib while you have company. People will be less likely to hold or pick up your baby if she is sleeping soundly. Consider planning a time of day to receive guests so you don't have a steady stream of people coming in and out of the house all day; if you can schedule people in advance, you'll be able to manage your sleeping and feeding times more comfortably. Planning the flow of visitors and helpful grandparents—so as not to overwhelm you or your baby—is an ideal task for your partner.

Q. I'm worried about my baby getting sick. Should visitors wear a mask?

A. Unless your visitor has a known infectious condition, do not be worried about exposing your baby to some normal germs. Of course, visitors should wash their hands with soap and water prior to touching your baby and avoid kissing him on the face. Newborns do not usually get sick—because they have a boost of maternal immunities and breastfed babies have even more protection. However, anyone who has a cold or a cough should not be around the baby because airborne droplets can be inhaled.

Q. My mother is visiting and I appreciate the help, but all she wants to do is hold the baby. I'm left doing all the chores when all I really want to do is be with my baby. Am I being ungrateful or should I say something?

A. Yes, you need to speak up and convey your feelings. It is important that you rest, not run around the house doing chores if there is another capable adult in the house. That person will not be there to take care of your baby in the middle of the night, and you will need your energy then. Don't be shy about asking for help at this time. Of course grandparents want to "ooh and ahh" over your bundle of joy, but it is not unreasonable to ask any visitor either to bring a meal or, at a minimum, not expect you to entertain them when they do visit. If you feel that you can't confront the grandparents in question, this is a great opportunity for your partner to speak up.

Q. Things were so easy in the hospital, but now I feel like I don't know what to *do* with my baby. All I do is watch him. What should I be doing?

A. Many new parents feel a similar sense of anticlimax upon arriving home. For the first few weeks, your new baby will sleep, eat, and cry—and likely not much else. That is why this stage is sometimes called the "babymoon" stage.

Take advantage of this time to take care of yourself, relax, and adjust to your new life. When the baby is sleeping it is a good idea to sleep, rest, shower, or eat something. Just make sure your baby is in a safe sleeping position, and never fall asleep on the couch with your baby.

It is not necessary to actively play with or overly stimulate your baby at this stage—you will be doing that in no time! Interact at this stage with your baby with plenty of cuddles, and sing or speak softly. To reiterate: what you and your baby really need is time to rest, eat, and relax. Keep in mind that the birthing process was tiring for your baby, too!

Q. I'm afraid to fall asleep because I feel like I won't hear my baby when she needs me. What happens if she spits up while we're both sleeping?

A. Many new parents I meet at the hospital feel exactly the same way, but try to relax and enjoy your sleep. Your baby will be fine! Most babies will turn their heads if they do spit up, so you don't have to worry. If your baby is sleeping, try your best to go to sleep, too, and if she needs to be fed or changed, there's no doubt you will hear her request! I can't emphasize enough that the best thing you can do for your baby is to take good care of yourself.

Baby Care Basics

Your health-care providers at the hospital will no doubt run through baby care with you before you are discharged, but it can feel a little unnerving once you're home and doing these things on your own for the first time.

Umbilical Cord

Your baby's umbilical cord will fall off within two to three weeks of delivery. It may be a little unsightly and will soon change color—white, yellow, and then black. Until it disappears, try to keep the area clean and dry. Fold your baby's diapers below the cord stump or choose diapers with that area cut out. It's best to keep the area exposed to the air and not under a wet diaper. You may notice a small amount of blood on the diaper when the cord finally does fall off, which is normal.

You may want to avoid giving your baby a tub bath until the cord has fallen off, and give him a sponge bath instead. If you do get the area wet, just make sure to dry it thoroughly. When the weather is warm, keep your baby in just a diaper and a T-shirt to help the area dry out. If your baby's T-shirts snap on the bottom, make sure that they're not too tight so they don't rub against the cord. Whether or not to use rubbing alcohol depends on your preference and that of your baby's pediatrician. Cleaning the area once or twice a day with alcohol on a cotton swab or pad is fine, but studies have found that letting the cord dry out naturally may be more effective.

Circumcision Care

If you have your baby boy circumcised, your nurse or health-care provider will show you how to care for his penis afterward. One of the most important things you need to do is keep the area clean. At every diaper change, use warm water and a cloth to gently wipe away any stool that may have come in contact with the area. Avoid bathing and using soaps or baby wipes for about a week to ten days, or until the wound is healed. Some pediatricians recommend wrapping the penis in gauze covered with petroleum jelly, or just applying a generous amount of petroleum jelly to the penis so that it doesn't stick to the diaper.

baby care tip

In addition to applying petroleum jelly to your baby's penis, smear some on the front of the diaper to prevent it from sticking. As the penis heals, it may develop a yellow crust or you may find a bit of blood on your baby's diaper—don't worry, this is all part of the healing process. Call your pediatrician if you notice redness around the normal skin, persistent bleeding, swelling, discharge, or a foul odor.

Changing Diapers

Make no mistake—after a few diaper changes, you'll be a pro at this baby ritual. Make sure you have all of the necessary supplies on hand before you begin. If your baby has a bowel movement, make sure you wipe from the front of your baby's bottom toward the back to prevent the spread of infection, and clean the stool from the folds in your baby's skin.

Your baby will inevitably cry for the first several weeks when you change her diaper. Most of the time she cries because she's cold or would just rather not be stirred. Soon enough, those diaper changing moments won't be a struggle but instead second nature—not to mention a great time for play and laughs with your baby.

baby care tip

When changing your newborn's diaper, he may perform a surprise urination or bowel movement while you're trying to get the clean diaper on or grab another wipe. This is in response to his bottom getting chilled when exposed to the air. To help avoid a mess, and to make changing in general quicker and easier, try sliding an open clean diaper under your baby's bottom and pulling a few wipes out before you take off the dirty diaper. Then, once your baby is clean, you can simply pull out the dirty diaper and quickly fasten the clean one—ideally keeping you clean and dry in the process!

PREVENTING DIAPER RASH

- Change your baby's diaper frequently (right away for stool diapers) in the first month. There will be a lot of both wet and dirty diapers during these weeks, so it will seem like you're changing diapers all the time! But by month two, this will slow down.
- Wipe your baby well and make sure any stool is cleaned off baby's bottom and leg creases.
- Use unscented wipes or plain water to clean your baby's bottom.
- If your baby's skin is sensitive, use an ointment on his bottom. There are two types of ointment: One is a barrier cream (such as A+D Ointment), which can be used after every diaper change. This cream will coat your baby's bottom and create a bit of a barrier between skin and stool. The other type of cream, usually white, contains zinc oxide. For babies who have some type of rash already, use cream with zinc oxide.

Q. Does it matter what types of wipes I choose for my baby?

A. Choose diaper wipes that are hypoallergenic and fragrance-free. For the first few weeks, it's a good idea to clean your baby's bottom with warm water and soap using a washcloth or paper towel; I have seen babies get a diaper rash from even the mildest wipes.

baby care tip

Baby wipes are pretty large, and most of us waste more than half of the wipe. To avoid waste, cut the rectangular wipes in half so that you have two small triangles. You can also use paper towels (ideally 100 percent recycled) cut into squares and moistened with a little warm water for your newborn's sensitive skin. Washcloths are also good; just try to embrace the laundry!

Q. My grandmother keeps telling me I should be using baby powder on my baby to keep him dry. Is this still true?

A. No—do not use baby powder around your baby for at least the first year, if not longer. The use of baby powder started many years ago when the only diapers available were very nonabsorbent cloth diapers. Because babies' bottoms were always wet, parents applied powder to help keep their babies dry. Diapers these days, both cloth and disposable, are so absorbent that babies' bottoms generally stay dry. Researchers have discovered that certain particles from baby powder that float in the air are actually harmful to babies and can lead to possible breathing problems. Researchers have also linked talcum powder to cervical cancer. So if you must use powder, wait until your baby is a year old and make sure it is cornstarch based.

Bathing

Q. How often should I bathe my newborn?

A. Babies do not need to be bathed every day. Every two to three days is fine during these early months when your baby will not get really dirty. Simply wiping your baby with a warm washcloth to clean her neck (where milk, formula, or spit-up tend to gather) and bottom once a day is usually all that is needed. Your baby has natural skin oils that will be washed away by too many baths.

In addition, it doesn't matter what time of the day you bathe your baby during the first month at home. Morning, afternoon, or night— she will adapt to the different times of day. When your baby is around two months old, bathing can become part of the bedtime routine if you choose. Nighttime routines that include baths help some babies transition from day to night mode. Just be sure to apply lotion afterward if you notice her skin getting dry from regular bathing.

Q. Do I need to purchase a separate shampoo and body wash?

A. No. In fact, one of the easiest ways to go more natural is to buy fewer products for your baby. One mild, hypoallergenic cleansing product is really all that is needed to wash your baby's skin and hair.

Q. I have never bathed a baby. How do I go about it?

A. The process of bathing your infant may seem complicated, but after you've done it a few times, it will start to come easy. Start by making sure you have all of the supplies you need handy, and add a few inches of lukewarm water to your infant tub. Your baby's head and ears should be far above water at all times.

Always test the water on the inside of your arm before placing your baby in the tub or check the temperature with a thermometer to ensure it's not warmer than 100 degrees (some baths come with a built-in thermometer and many bath toys have them, too). Undress your baby while talking softly to him and take off his diaper. Gently pick him up by supporting the back of his neck and head with one hand, and cradle his bottom with your other hand and lower arm. Slowly lower your baby's feet into the water followed by the rest of his body. It's perfectly normal for your baby to cry—just keep talking to him in a calm and soothing voice while you wash him up.

Especially during the first month, there's no need to use soap on your baby's face. Wiping his eyes, nose, mouth, and forehead with a wet washcloth will do the trick. Use a small dab of soap to wash your baby's hair once a week and don't be afraid to scrub with your fingertips. Massaging your baby's head actually gets circulation going and can help alleviate cradle cap. To rinse, fill a container (preferably one with a pour spout) with clean, lukewarm water and pour it slowly onto your baby's head, making sure not to allow water to run down his face. If you do spill a bit onto the face, just wipe it away with a dry cloth.

Then use a thin washcloth (or just your hands, if you prefer) to get in-between your baby's tiny toes and fingers—you'd be surprised at how easy it is to forget about those little crevices and how much can build up there! Other areas you should cover include the underarms, bottom, genitals, behind the ears, under the chin, and around the neck, legs, arms, back, and belly button. Be sure to rinse the soap off thoroughly. If you're using your hands, rub a small amount of soap in your hands and get into all of the crevices—that way your baby will likely love the massage!

When you're done, place your hands firmly under your baby's armpits, cupping your fingers around the sides of his body. Slowly raise your baby up and gently place him down onto a clean, dry towel and pat dry.

BATH-TIME DOS AND DON'TS

- Don't fill the bathtub while your baby is in the tub.
- Don't leave your baby's side while she is in the tub.
- Do warm up the bathroom beforehand.
- Do test the water on the inside of your arm or with a thermometer before placing your infant into the tub.
- Do place a warm washcloth on the larger air-exposed areas of your baby's skin to help keep her warm during bath time. Because your baby's belly, for example, will likely be sticking out of the water, her skin may chill and make her cry.

baby care tip

When giving your infant a bath, start out by warming up the bathroom. You can do this by turning up the heat ten minutes before bath time, turning on the bathroom heat fan if you have one, or bringing in a space heater and putting it in a safe place away from water and your baby. Providing a warm-air environment will likely minimize cries due to being cold before and after the bath.

Skin, Nail, and Dental Care

During the first few months, do not use clippers or scissors on your baby's nails even if they appear long enough to cut. Babies' nails adhere to the skin on the fingertips, so in order to avoid accidently nicking your baby's skin, use an emery board very gently to file down the nails if your baby is scratching himself. If the long nails don't bother your baby, then leave them alone—they will eventually begin to break off. Another option is to dress your baby in T-shirts that have hand covers or mitts to prevent an accidental scratch.

> ### baby care tip
> If your baby scratches himself with his nails, rub a few drops of breast milk on the cut. When applied topically, breast milk helps prevent infection and promotes healing by fighting off bacteria and viruses.

Q. Does my baby need lotion or moisturizer?

A. That depends. Almost all babies are born with skin that looks dry around the hands, feet, and ankles—a normal result of being surrounded by amniotic fluid for nine months. This layer of skin will flake off during the first few weeks of life, and moisturizers will not speed the process. As your newborn gets older, though, if his skin continues to get dry or develop eczema then moisturizing it will help. Babies are especially prone to eczema and dry skin in the winter months. Ask your pediatrician what she recommends for treating dry skin conditions.

> ### baby care tip
> If you're looking for a moisturizer for your baby, think about using jojoba oil. I love this oil because it provides moisture for the skin all day long, has great nutritional properties, and allows the skin to breathe. A small amount will go a long way. It's a bit more expensive than traditional baby oils, but it lasts a long time and the organic variety is free of pesticides.

Q. Can I use sunscreen on my newborn?

A. Try to avoid using sunscreen on your infant until she is at least six months old. Babies have very thin, delicate skin, which leads to increased absorption of chemicals. Try to shield her from the harmful rays of the sun by dressing her in protective, lightweight clothing and using an umbrella. If you are heading to the beach or are worried about sun exposure, check with your baby's pediatrician about sunscreen use.

Q. I've heard that I should brush my baby's teeth and gums. Is it safe to use toothpaste?

A. No, your baby should not have toothpaste. Simply wipe your baby's gums occasionally with a wet washcloth. Even when teeth start coming in, which may be as early as three months, it is fine to wipe them or use a very soft toothbrush specifically designed for baby teeth. When your baby gets older, check with your pediatrician for recommendations regarding fluoride and toothpaste.

Vaccinations

Q. My pediatrician has recommended that my baby gets her scheduled vaccines next month at her next checkup. Are these vaccines safe?

A. Immunizing our children is no different from any of the other ways we protect them from harm. It can be a very controversial subject. These days we are bombarded with information from many sources, which is often frustratingly contradictory. Despite the controversies, the success of immunization over the past fifty years is astonishing. As in the recent outbreak of measles due to decreased immunization, we will start to see diseases emerge that had been considered eradicated if this trend continues.

When making decisions about immunizing our children, we must consider the sources from which we are getting our information. Anyone can put anything online—whether it's true or not! The very best source of information is your child's doctor. Most pediatricians commit their careers to keeping kids safe and healthy. Recommending the immunization guidelines from the American Academy of Pediatrics is one of the most important ways to do that. If you want to do further research, ask your physician to direct you to Web sites that are based on verified scientific knowledge and research, such as the CDC Web site (cdc.gov).

There is a lot of false information out there about dangers of immunizing children, most of which has been proven to be incorrect based on scientific research. There is a common myth that the MMR (measles, mumps, and rubella) vaccine causes autism. This theory has been closely studied and is simply not true. All thimerosal (a mercury preservative previously used in immunizations) has been removed, despite clear evidence that this preservative was never associated with harm in children. The examples go on and on. Just like we educate ourselves about the safety of different car seats, cribs, and mattresses, we must be sure to properly educate ourselves about immunizations from reliable sources.

We all have a part in protecting our children. The more kids who are immunized in your community, the less likely it is that your own children will be exposed to disease. It's like a four-way intersection. Every now and then a car can sneak through the intersection without stopping, but if everyone went through without stopping, chaos would result and people would get hurt. Just as we are sure to stop at a stop sign while our children are safely buckled in the back seat of our car, we must stop and think about the importance of fully immunizing our kids for their benefit and the benefit of others.

Feeding

Again, one of your baby's goals during the first two weeks is to regain the weight she may have lost in the hospital. Most breastfed newborns lose 5 to 8 percent of their body weight in their first few days, and some lose up to 10 percent. This is fine as long as your baby starts to gain weight steadily during the first two weeks. If your baby loses 10 percent or more, your pediatrician may recommend a supplement (see chapter 9) along with close monitoring of your baby's weight. Most pediatricians like to see babies at their birth weight or above at the two-week office visit. Bottle-fed babies, on the other hand, usually do not lose weight, and if they do it is generally back on within a few days.

If you are bottle-feeding your baby, it is relatively easy to establish a flexible feeding schedule. Most babies at this age take between two and four ounces of formula per feeding. Feeding your baby every three to four hours will give her enough time between feedings to digest her food. Feeding too frequently will get your baby in the habit of snacking and dozing instead of eating and sleeping. If your baby fusses between feedings, you may want to offer a pacifier to help soothe and calm her. Giving her a pacifier now does not mean your baby will be walking around with a pacifier when she is four years old. Once her need for sucking diminishes (at approximately four months), you may find it is time to get rid of the pacifier. While your baby may miss it for a few days, at this early age habits are easy to break. Of course, if you're following AAP recommendations for reducing the risk of SIDS, it's not a problem to keep using the pacifier for the first year.

Breastfeeding

Q. Help—I'm exhausted! My ten-day-old baby is constantly breastfeeding. He only feeds for a few minutes and then falls asleep, but when I take him off of the breast he wakes up and fusses. What can I do to keep him awake while feeding?

A. This is a common dilemma new breastfeeding moms face during the first few weeks. Some sleepy babies need to be woken up frequently during a feeding session. When you first start to breastfeed your baby, make sure he is wide awake—even crying. Latch your baby onto the breast and continue to stimulate him during the feeding session. It is normal for a baby to pause during a feed, but try to keep the pauses short. Count to five and if your baby does not resume sucking then rub his back, tickle his feet, or massage his hands until he wakes up and resumes. Keep feeding and occasionally compress and massage your breasts so that the milk flows more easily into your baby's mouth.

Try to breastfeed for a minimum of fifteen to twenty minutes at a time. If he begins vigorously sucking, he can remain on one breast for up to thirty minutes. Offer the second breast to your baby, but first try to wake and stimulate again. You may even need to change his diaper—this movement (and the cold wipe) will help your baby wake up again. Re-latch him to the opposite breast and continue the feeding session. Continue with the waking techniques described above until your baby has fed for at least another fifteen minutes. When your baby is finished feeding, gently burp him, swaddle him, and place him into his bassinet or crib to sleep. Your baby will start to feed much better when you use the waking techniques. He may even sleep for up to three hours between feedings, and when he wakes up he will be rested and hungry enough to feed for longer periods of time.

FORMULA FEEDING

There are several formula-feeding options on the market today, and all of those manufactured in the United States must pass strict nutritional standards set by the FDA. Here is an overview of the types you can choose.

- Cow's milk–based formula (organic and non-organic): Makes up the majority of the formulas on the market. Most are fortified with iron, which is recommended by the AAP.

- Soy milk–based formula: Sometimes recommended for babies allergic to cow's-milk protein. However, many babies who are allergic to the cow's-milk protein may also be allergic to the protein in soy. If your baby does not tolerate cow's milk–based formula or soy, he will need another formula. Consult your baby's pediatrician for appropriate options and brands.

- Hypoallergenic formula: For babies who are allergic to both cow's milk- and soy-based formulas. This formula comes with the protein partially broken down so the baby can digest it more easily.

- Specialized formula: These formulas are usually fed to preterm or low-birth-weight babies because they have more calories than standard formulas.

Q. Should I feed my baby with soy- or milk-based formula? Can I switch from one to the other?

A. Keep your baby on the same formula that was offered in the hospital, which is usually a fortified milk-based formula. Most hospitals use brands that are readily available to purchase in stores. Do not casually switch formulas. If it seems like your baby is not tolerating the formula, or seems very gassy, contact your pediatrician before switching to a soy-based formula or a hypoallergenic brand. It sometimes takes up to a week for a baby to get used to a new formula, so give it some time. Most pediatricians recommend that parents start their baby out on a milk-based formula fortified with iron.

Q. What is the difference between the types of formula?

A. There are three basic types of formula to choose from: powder, concentrate, and ready-to-use. The powder form, which is mixed with water, is the least expensive. Concentrates must be diluted with water before using. Ready-to-use formula can be poured right from the container and fed to your baby—no mixing or measuring required. This is a convenient option but more expensive.

baby care tip

When using powdered formula, you don't have to worry about keeping it cool or refrigerated. Just throw some water bottles in your diaper bag, and when you're ready to feed your baby add the water to the bottle. Mix in the appropriate amount of powder, shake, and you are ready to feed.

Q. What are the DHA and ARA in infant formula? Does my baby need these?

A. DHA stands for docosahexaenoic acid and ARA stands for arachidonic acid. These are polyunsaturated (good) fatty acids linked to numerous health benefits including brain, vision, and nerve development in infants. These fats are naturally found in many foods, including eggs and fish oils, and because they are also found in breast milk, manufacturers add DHA and ARA to formula in attempts to make it more like breast milk. Current research has not yet concluded whether or not these actually benefit an infant's cognitive development.

Q. I am lactose-intolerant—does this mean my baby is also likely to be lactose-intolerant? If so, should I start him on soy formula?

A. No, it is highly unlikely that your baby will also be lactose-intolerant. Lactose is a sugar that is found in all milks including human, cow, and goat. Most babies have an enzyme, called lactase, that breaks down this sugar. It is the cow's-milk proteins that cause tummy distress in some babies, and sometimes switching to a soy-based formula may help. Just talk to your baby's pediatrician before making this decision.

> ## baby care tip
>
> If you have expressed breast milk and want to transition to formula, mix some breast milk with some formula so your baby's system can slowly get used to it.

Q. I am formula-feeding my baby. What types of bottles and nipples should I buy?

A. There are many different types of bottles on the market and your baby will feed just fine from any of them. If you choose plastic, just make sure it is BPA-free, as most bottles on the market are nowadays. Opt for a silicone (clear) nipple instead of latex (brown) rubber if possible. Silicone nipples last longer and latex allergies are becoming more and more common. Also, you will want to make sure that you choose the size that reflects your baby's age. Newborns need a slow flow nipple so make sure you choose a newborn size (or stage one). As your baby grows he will want a faster flow (typically by three months but he may demand it sooner!). If your baby seems frustrated because it is taking too long for him to feed then it may be time to get him a nipple with a slightly faster flow.

> ## baby care tip
>
> The good old-fashioned method of a mild (or organic) dish soap and water is the best way to clean your baby's bottles and nipples daily. You will need a bottle brush to clean hard-to-reach spots in the bottle. It's fine to put the bottle in the dishwasher if you prefer, but do not put the nipples in the dishwasher (or microwave). Constantly exposing plastics to high temperatures will cause them to break down.

Q. How often should I burp my baby?

A. Bottle-fed babies—whether it's formula or breast milk in the bottle—should be burped more frequently than directly breastfed babies because more air is taken in through the artificial nipple. A good rule of thumb is to burp your baby after every one to two ounces during the first two weeks. Taking a pause to burp mid-feed will help reduce the air buildup that may cause your baby to spit up. You can burp in several different positions:

- Sit your baby upright on your lap and support his chin and neck with one hand while patting his back with the other. This can also help wake your baby up so he can get in a good feeding.

- Rest your baby upright on your chest, with his chin at your shoulder. Just keep in mind that your baby may try to lift his head up, and with so little head control could easily bump himself on your shoulder. (And if snuggled too close on your chest, your baby may tend to go right to sleep instead of continuing the feeding.)

- If your baby is not too prone to spitting up, another option is to lay him belly down across your lap and gently rub or pat his back.

If your baby starts to fuss at the bottle or spits the bottle out, you may want to try to burp him before finishing the feeding. Burp for about a minute. If nothing comes up, you're done.

Breastfed babies don't get much air while eating, so don't try to take your baby off the breast to burp unless he really needs it. Your baby may be indicating that he needs to be burped if he starts to get fussy at the breast and doesn't want to continue a feeding.

Sleeping

As mentioned in chapter 9, your baby's biological clock will not begin to mature until about six to nine weeks of age. During this period she may prefer to sleep during the day and be up at night. The good news is that for the first two weeks, when your baby does wake up at night, she will likely go right back to sleep after a feeding.

Most newborns sleep up to sixteen hours per day. During the day it's a good idea to wake your baby every two to two and a half hours for a feeding if you're breastfeeding and every three to three and a half hours if you're bottle-feeding. By waking your baby you are sending her signals that daytime is wake time and nighttime is sleep time. Most babies have one long sleep stretch of about four hours (maybe five if bottle-feeding) during this stage, but do not let your baby sleep this long during the day. Try to save the long stretch for a time that is convenient for you, perhaps midnight to four in the morning.

During the initial daytime sleep spells, take advantage and get some rest for yourself. Don't send thank-you notes, prepare meals, or clean the house. Rest in your bed, or at least relax and read a book or magazine.

Q. Should we use a nightlight in our baby's room at night?

A. This is a personal choice. There really is no compelling reason to use a nightlight in your baby's room, especially when she is under the age of two (babies this age typically do not suffer from nightmares and are not afraid of the dark). Your baby may actually sleep better in a completely darkened room. If you decide to use a nightlight, choose one that provides low lighting and place it away from your baby. Also make sure that the nightlight is not touching or placed near any fabric such as comforters, blankets, or curtains.

baby care tip

While your baby doesn't need a nightlight, having one in her room may be helpful if you need to feed in the middle of the night. It's certainly better to use a dim nightlight than to completely brighten the room. This will help to keep your baby (and you!) in a somewhat drowsy state.

Q. My baby sleeps through the night. Should I wake her every three hours to feed her?

A. This depends on whether or not your baby is gaining weight. Most pediatricians will recommend waking your baby to feed every three hours until your baby has regained his birth weight. Breastfed babies need nine to twelve feeds in a twenty-four-hour period, so feed your baby often during the day. If she is gaining weight, you should not have to wake her more than once during the night for a feed; most likely she will wake up on her own to feed at least once, maybe twice. It may sound tiring but this can be a good thing, especially at first, because breastfeeding at night helps to keep up your milk supply.

Bottle-fed babies tend to sleep for longer stretches. Ideally a baby will eat often during the day and have one long sleep stretch at night, perhaps between three and five hours. If your baby is not gaining weight or is slow to gain weight, it is important to feed him at least once during the night. Your baby needs those extra calories.

Soothing

During the first several weeks at home, most babies are generally not fussy yet and are easily soothed. They tend to be relatively easy to care for, mostly eating and sleeping. When they cry it is often due to hunger, so it generally subsides with a full tummy. But if your baby's tummy is full and his diaper is clean, his cries or fusses may mean he needs some soothing. Usually just picking up and holding your baby will do the trick at this age—he will probably calm right down and fall asleep. If your baby needs a little more than just being held try a few different soothing techniques.

BABY CARE TECHNIQUES TO SOOTHE YOUR BABY

- Make sure your baby's basic needs are met, including feeding, changing the diaper, burping, and making sure clothing is not too tight and your baby is not too hot or cold. Also consider whether or not he may just be very tired and need some sleep.
- Offer your baby a finger or pacifier to suck on.
- Hold your baby on his side and walk around the house with a little bounce in your step. Babies love rhythmic movement, and this simple motion might calm him right down. Be sure to cradle his head carefully.
- Swaddle your baby.
- Place your baby in a bouncy seat, with or without a swaddle. Try turning the vibration on if your seat comes with the option.
- Turn on a white-noise machine.
- Place your baby in a swing. However, if he's really upset, try to calm him down a bit first by rocking and bouncing him gently. Stay close to him for a few minutes to ease the transition.

- Put on some relaxing music.
- Take your baby outside for a walk in the stroller.
- Place your baby in a sling or front carrier and walk around your house or go outside for a walk.
- Take your baby out for a ride in the car.

baby care tip

Consider joining a new moms' group to learn more soothing techniques and share your experiences. It will be nice to find out that other moms are going through the same things with their newborns.

If none of your soothing efforts work, simply place your baby in a safe place (such as a crib) and let him cry for a while. Check on him every five to ten minutes to make sure he's all right. If you can, call a friend, neighbor, or family member to come over and relieve you for a bit. The key is to be patient, take regular deep breaths, and count to ten when you feel frustrated. Remember, this too shall pass—most babies will outgrow their crying spells within a few weeks.

baby care tip

When you find you have tried everything and your baby is still crying, take him out for a ride—he may fall asleep in the car. Then find the nearest drive-through so you can get yourself a cup of coffee or a snack.

Soothing Tools

THE PACIFIER

Q. My baby had a pacifier in the hospital. Will this affect his ability to breastfeed?

A. Probably not, but now that you're home it's a good idea to wait a few weeks before reintroducing a pacifier until breastfeeding is fully established.

The research on nipple confusion indicates that most babies do not confuse a pacifier with breastfeeding (it's usually bottle nipples that can interfere). The jaw-tongue action required to suck and hold a pacifier in the mouth is different from the movements needed to get milk out of a breast. They are different skills. Sometimes a pacifier can even reinforce good sucking behavior. Some lactation consultants are strict about not using a pacifier, but research shows that we can ease up on these worries a bit. If your baby has the need to suck in order to be soothed, offer him the pacifier. If he has a hard time going back onto the breast, then try avoiding the pacifier for a few days. Trying the pacifier will do no harm—you can always decide if it is helpful or not.

PACIFIER DOS AND DON'TS

As I discussed in chapter 2, for SIDS-prevention reasons, the American Academy of Pediatrics recommends the use of pacifiers at nap time and bedtime throughout the first year of life. However, it is recommended that pacifier introduction for breastfed infants be delayed for the first two to three weeks to ensure that breastfeeding is firmly established. In addition, if your infant refuses the pacifier, it should not be forced into his mouth. Forcing a pacifier will make the baby push it out of his mouth with his tongue, defeating the soothing purpose of it. Gently rub your baby's lips with the pacifier and wait for him to be interested enough to draw it into his mouth. Some other tips for effective pacifier use include:

- Let your baby decide. Some babies are not interested in pacifiers, and this is no cause for concern. If your baby isn't, try soothing him another way (rocking, singing, letting him suck on the tip of your pinky finger). Just don't let your breast or the bottle become the pacifier.

- Buy one-piece pacifiers. Two-piece pacifiers or those with a small plastic handle can be a safety risk if they break. Find a one-piece style your baby likes and buy some backups. Once your baby has decided which pacifier suits him, be brand-loyal.

- Be careful with pacifier clips. Many such clips come with long straps, but you should use only short straps that can't get caught around your baby's neck.

baby care tip

Use mild dish soap and warm water to thoroughly clean your baby's new pacifier before giving it to him. Make sure to regularly clean it (and really dig into and wash any crevices). As time goes on, watch the pacifier to see if it starts to look faded and worn out, and then replace as necessary. You'll also know it's time to throw one out when it becomes "tacky" to the touch. This is a sign of rubber degradation and, if ignored, can lead to the pacifier becoming a choking hazard as the rubber nipple can break off.

THE SWADDLE

Most babies under three months are soothed by the sensations of being wrapped up in a blanket or swaddle cloth, as it mimics the secure, compact feeling of the womb. Try swaddling your baby with his arms at his sides, and then walk around with him. You don't want to give up on swaddling right away. If your baby is crying and doesn't calm down, keep him swaddled, offer a pacifier or finger to suck on, and continue to walk around the house. It is usually not the swaddle that makes babies unhappy but the motions of the swaddling process.

Make sure you learn an easy and effective swaddle technique before you leave the hospital with your baby. If your baby is too sleepy during the day, try swaddling him more loosely and leave his hands free. That way he is more likely to wake himself up for feedings. If your baby is more active and awake at night or during the evening, swaddle him a bit tighter with his hands down so he can get a good stretch of uninterrupted sleep. It is well worth repeating that your baby should only be placed *on his back* while swaddled—never on his stomach or side. When your baby starts rolling over, swap the swaddle for something that keeps his arms free, such as a wearable sleep sack.

Q. Why will swaddling help to soothe my baby?

A. Swaddling and sucking are the two most important soothers that will calm and relax your baby during the first few months. Because her nervous system is still highly immature, swaddling her securely in a light blanket can help give her a sense of comfort and security— again, much like the feeling she had in the womb.

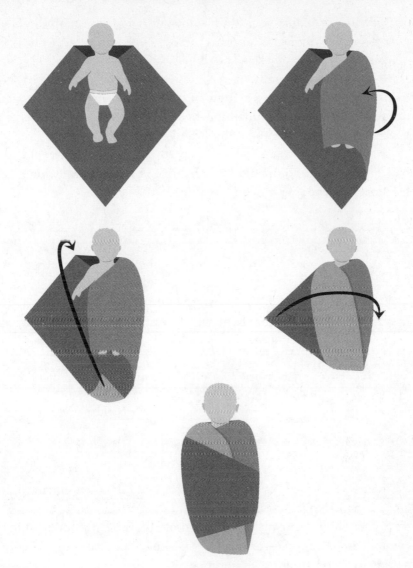

FIGURE 10-1: How to swaddle a baby

When you first try swaddling it may seem as though your baby does not want to be wrapped up (due to her protests), but I highly recommend you keep trying it. You have a better idea than your baby does of what is best for her, so fight that urge to give up if she fusses initially. You can even try swaddling her when she's not fussy (before a nap, for example). The more she gets used to it, the better a tool the swaddle will be in soothing her.

Swaddle as long as your baby enjoys it, at least through the first twelve weeks. The key to a good swaddle is using a large-enough blanket or appropriately sized swaddle cloth so it stays wrapped even when she moves. It's important to always keep the top edge of the blanket under your baby's chin to avoid trapping air near the mouth (or rebreathing) and, as I mentioned, always place your baby on her back to sleep (with or without the swaddle).

Q. **I feel like I'm squishing my baby. Aren't I taking away his freedom by wrapping him up like this?**

A. You are not denying your baby his freedom by swaddling him. On the contrary, your baby craves the feeling of security and comfort that swaddling provides. You may not need to swaddle your baby at all in the daytime for soothing purposes, but when it's time to sleep at night, swaddle him snugly. Your baby's Moro reflex (also known as the "startle reflex") causes him to make sudden involuntary jerky movements that, while sleeping, can cause him to awaken. This reflex can last up to and even after three to four months of age, but swaddling will reduce this unnecessary disruption and allow you and your baby to get a more consistent night's sleep.

Development
. . . .

In order to best care for your baby it is helpful to understand her developmental level at birth and during the first month at home. At birth your baby is already learning about and noticing things in her environment. Her senses are all very well developed, so she can begin getting used to her new surroundings.

Q. **What can my baby see during her first month?**

A. At birth your baby can make out lights, shapes, and movements from about eight to fifteen inches away. But babies don't have peripheral vision, and can only focus on one thing at a time, so make sure you position yourself in front of your baby's eyes so she can see and study you. Your baby also sees contrasting colors, and within a few weeks she will become particularly interested in bold, black-and-white images. A contrasting pattern on a mobile will keep your baby's attention and stimulate her sense of vision.

> ## baby care tip
>
> If your baby was born preterm or has some feeding concerns, expect your pediatrician to pay particular attention to your baby's growth, development, and feeding patterns.

Q. What can my baby hear?

A. Your baby's sense of hearing will develop while he is still in utero. At birth, your baby will be able to hear voices and may well even respond to the familiar sound of your voice.

Babies love language, so it is important to speak to your baby when he is awake and playing. Newborns can even absorb language just by listening to others speak, so having your baby around you, listening to regular conversation, is good for him. Babies are also calmed by music—a language of sorts. Listening to soothing music at regular wind-down times in the day can be calming for your baby and can help to set up a routine that will help him soothe himself as he gets older.

Q. What can I do to stimulate my baby's sense of touch?

A. Your baby will love everyday events such as feeling the water in his bath, being massaged, and spending lots of skin-to-skin time with both parents. As he gets older you can experiment with different textures and get creative, but right now he is just getting used to you and the world around him.

Q. Does my baby really know my smell?

A. Yes, your baby will be able to taste and smell to some extent from the time he is born. Researchers have found that the senses of smell and taste are linked and that a newborn is capable of recognizing the scent of his mother.[38] So hold your baby close—he'll love it!

---

38 N. Rones, "Your Baby's Developing Senses," *Parents*, parents.com/baby/development/physical/babies-developing-senses.

Milestones

At your one-month pediatrician appointment, your baby's health-care provider will perform a physical exam on your baby, assess your baby's weight, height, and head circumference, ask about your baby's sleeping and eating patterns, and address any concerns you have. Around the end of the first month your baby be may able to:

- Lift his head for a few seconds at a time while on his stomach
- Follow objects with his eyes
- Respond to sounds
- Stare at faces and contrasting objects
- Grasp strongly

Your First Month as a Mom

. . . .

The hospital stay may have offered you a short chance to rest while the nurses were on hand to help, but you still need to focus on resting and recovering when you get home. You may feel a rush of adrenaline during the first week home, but this will wear off and the need to nap will eventually win out. The cliché "Sleep when your baby sleeps" is really a good rule of thumb. Sleep is critical to your recovery and helps you to maintain a sense of well-being. It is normal for you to feel anxious about your new responsibilities, and elevated hormone levels can add to an overly emotional state. Take things slow, rest when you can, and eat a balanced diet, which should include six small meals per day. Keep your water glass filled and drink every time you feed your baby. Your body has just completed one of life's amazing wonders and needs time to rest.

In terms of physical appearance, when you arrive home you may still look and feel about seven months pregnant. Many new moms don't lose many pounds during birth due to various factors like intravenous fluids and new milk production, which make your breasts fuller. For some women, it's common to weigh the same going home as they weighed when they went in for labor. Many women will also continue to see the linea negra, a vertical brownish line on the front of the abdomen, for another three to nine months. Do yourself a favor and don't get on the scale yet. Give yourself a few weeks to recover and let your body adjust.

Q. My bottom is really painful and it hurts to walk around and get up from a chair, among other things. Is that normal?

A. Yes, pain after birth is normal, especially if you had an episiotomy or vaginal tear or have hemorrhoids. Although it may be uncomfortable, do some Kegel exercises, which will help heal the perineum by promoting circulation and increasing blood flow.

For the first few days at home, you may find relief in taking a sitz bath in the morning and at night (your nurse will give you the plastic device to take home). You may also find relief by applying a cold compress or ice pack to your bottom (put some crushed ice in a zip-top bag and wrap a towel around it), which helps reduce swelling. Topical creams and ointments from the hospital may help for a short time, too. Finally, wash with the hospital squirt bottle instead of wiping after using the bathroom. This will not only make the area feel a bit better but avoids unwanted friction. Taking approved pain medication will help you bear the few days of discomfort and then the worst of the pain will dissipate.

If you are suffering from hemorrhoids, as many new moms do, the best position to promote healing is to sit reclined on a doughnut-shaped pillow. You don't want gravity to put pressure on the bottom, and if you sit up for a long time you'll get sore. Your health-care provider can write you a prescription for a steroid cream if your hemorrhoids are not healing well. Make sure you are getting enough fiber in your diet, eating plenty of fresh fruits and vegetables, and drinking at least eight glasses (about a liter and a half) of water a day.

It's also important to get in a little bit of activity—a short walk outside, for example—to help increase blood circulation and promote healing. Don't overdo it, though; simple movement is all you need at this stage, once per day at most.

Q. Is it OK to take a bath in my first few days at home?

A. Talk to your health-care provider about when it is safe to take a bath—if you had a C-section, you'll want to avoid baths for a few weeks to prevent infection and allow time for healing. However, much like a sitz bath, taking a warm bath will relieve the discomfort you may feel from a vaginal tear, episiotomy, or hemorrhoids. It will also give you a few relaxing minutes by yourself!

AT HOME AFTER A C-SECTION

If you had a C-section, you should spend your first few days after birth reclined with pillows resting and healing. This is important because you may still be on pain medications and feel extremely tired. You should also try to avoid lifting—while you may of course pick up your baby when necessary, try to arrange to have someone bring her to you for cuddles and feedings while you are recovering.

Your milk may not come in for a few more days or even a week, in which case your baby will probably require some supplementation with formula. Enlist the help of Dad/Partner, friends, or family to assist you with this, as well as diapering, sponge baths, and keeping you well fed and hydrated. Visitors should only be there to help!

Q. I'm so tired— I expected to be exhausted but this is even more difficult than I anticipated. Will I always feel like this?

A. The first few weeks with a new baby can be tiring and overwhelming. You are recovering from birth, a process that can take between two to six weeks or sometimes even longer. Don't put pressure on yourself—take things slow. Your baby will sleep a lot during the first few weeks and your main job during this period is to sleep and rest yourself. Accept all of the help offered to you!

Q. I find myself getting teary and even crying more than usual. I feel overwhelmed—is this normal?

A. The "baby blues" affect 80 percent of new moms to varying degrees. They can strike anytime in the first few weeks. Some women feel very weepy, or find they laugh and cry at the same time. Considering the physical stresses of labor combined with the surge in hormones in your body, this is completely normal. The more sleep you can get, the better you will feel. Being tired makes everything feel overwhelming. These feelings can last up to two weeks, but if they continue without letting up after that, you should see your health-care provider. Remember that baby blues are not the same as postpartum depression. Based on the latest research, postpartum depression affects less than 20 percent of women. If you have two or more of the warning signs (see below), please see your physician as soon as possible. Treatment for postpartum depression is usually very effective.

I receive a lot of questions from parents about the difference between typical baby blues and postpartum depression (PPD). A worried new father called me recently with concerns because his wife had a family history of PPD and seemed to be showing some signs. I suggested it might be helpful for me to come to their home to educate them about PPD. Mom looked exhausted and clearly needed to get some rest. She expressed feeling like she was breastfeeding the baby all day long and had no time for anything else. I spent the afternoon teaching Mom a simple schedule for her two-week-old baby that gave her time to nap, shower, eat, and even watch television. It worked! Mom called me a few days later saying she was sleeping and had more time than ever. She actually started a scrapbook project she had put on hold for years. In this mom's case, she was feeling depressed but did not necessarily have PPD. She simply needed to identify how she felt and find a few solutions. But again, it's always better to call your health-care provider to check in if you experience any prolonged PPD symptoms.

WARNING SIGNS OF POSTPARTUM DEPRESSION (PPD)

Postpartum depression can be a concern and even debilitating for new mothers. It is important for both you and your spouse or partner to look out for these signs of PPD:

- "Baby blues" that don't seem to be going away
- Loss of interest in the baby. By this I don't just mean being too tired to feed the baby in the middle of the night, feeling like you want your partner to take over with the baby when he comes home from work, or feeling like you need a break. This warning sign relates to losing complete interest in responding to your baby in any way and feeling that you would rather be somewhere else without any desire to get back to your baby after a break.
- Inability to sleep
- Any feelings of violence toward the baby

Q. My partner wants to help with the baby but I want to be the one to do everything. What is wrong with me?

A. Don't worry, there is nothing wrong with you. The surge of hormones makes it hard for you to let anyone else do anything for your baby. It's normal to feel the urge to do everything and to want to be in control of your newborn. Keep in mind, however, that it is important (and very helpful to you) for Dad/Partner and baby to bond. That means changing diapers, giving bottles if bottle-feeding, baths, and cuddling. It is OK if he changes the baby differently than you do—slightly varying routines and systems are fine, and your entire family will reap the benefits of cohesively sharing in these experiences.

baby care tip

The role your baby's father plays in your day-to-day activities is largely influenced by your attitude. This is new territory for him, too, and he'll need plenty of encouragement from you. Tell him he's doing a great job, and support and appreciate his own ways of bonding with and caring for the baby.

Q. My husband took off one week but is returning to work now. Why am I so terrified of being alone with my baby?

A. Now is a great time to reach out to family members and/or friends and schedule times for visitors to come by during the day. It is normal to feel overwhelmed and scared, but remember, you are this baby's mother and you can do this. Look to my suggested schedules at the end of this chapter for ideas on how to structure your day. These schedules allow you to manage your time and your baby's schedule in the most efficient way possible to help you take the best care of both of you. Look into resources through your hospital or online for local mom-and-baby groups. You will want to get out a bit more in the next few weeks, and baby groups are a great way to meet other moms going through the same things you are.

MOM DOS AND DON'TS FOR FIRST MONTH

▶ **DO**
- Take the baby out for a walk in the stroller
- Get fresh air every day
- Order food for takeout or delivery
- Accept help from family and friends
- Rest as much as possible
- Snack on healthy foods during the day
- Sleep as much as you can, day or night

▶ **DON'T**
- Go grocery shopping or attempt to run any errands
- Clean your house or do any major cooking
- Lift or carry heavy objects
- Do household chores or laundry
- Work
- Write thank-you notes
- Worry about stimulating your baby

baby care tip

Thought it was difficult to get out the door before you had your baby? If you and your baby need to go somewhere, tack on an extra twenty or so minutes of planning time before you leave the house. Collecting all of the gear you'll need and preparing the diaper bag can take time, not to mention the unexpected, last-minute diaper change!

Don't leave home without:
- Weather appropriate blanket
- Weather-appropriate hat
- Pacifiers
- At least four diapers
- Container of wipes
- At least two Onesies-style bodysuits
- At least two one-piece pajamas
- Stroller or baby carrier, depending on your destination
- At least two burp cloths
- If bottle-feeding, bottles and enough formula for the time you'll be out (as well as clean water to mix with formula if your destination will not have it)
- If breastfeeding, breastfeeding cover or blanket and nursing pads

Right before you go, remember to:
- Feed your baby to maximize the happy, well-fed baby time you have while out
- Change your baby's diaper
- Make a list of errands you need to run or items you need to buy while out (it'll be disheartening to realize you forgot the one item you went out to get!)

Q. After a few days in the house I feel like I'm starting to go stir crazy. Is it OK to take my baby outside or to a public place?

A. Yes, fresh air is great for newborns as well as for parents. Take your baby for a walk in a stroller or a newborn-safe carrier, sling, or wrap. Most pediatricians recommend waiting until your baby has had one set of immunizations (two to six weeks) to expose him to very crowded public areas. Airplanes are usually fine once baby has had one set of immunizations.

It will be great for you physically and mentally to get outside and take a walk. This kind of gentle activity can help boost circulation, which will help with constipation and promote vaginal healing. But as I discussed earlier in the chapter, if you had a C-section you should take it easy at home for at least ten days before venturing on any major outings.

Checking in with Dad (or Partner)

Dads (or partners) can also feel overwhelmed by the new arrival in the family. Often they have feelings of anxiety and stress over how they are going to care for their new family. They can feel out of their element with regard to newborn care, and sometimes the extreme closeness of mom and baby can make dads/partners feel isolated and even jealous. These feelings will go away after things settle down a bit.

Some report feeling let down in the beginning. Because a breast-feeding mom is essentially the primary provider for a baby during the first few weeks, the other parent can feel deprived of ways to bond. But there are many ways for Dad/Partner to be involved with the baby these days—changing the baby's diapers, giving the baby massages, and physically connecting with the baby by just holding and cuddling him. Bottle-fed babies can also enjoy time with Dad/other parent during feedings, and this can be very rewarding for both!

Dads/Partners, one of the best ways to help your family during these early weeks is to make sure Mom is getting the support she needs. Be the "go-to" for any necessary store runs, prescription pick-ups, laundry, and nighttime feeding assistance. If you can take some time off work for this first stage, it will help lighten the load on Mom and make things go much more smoothly. As I mentioned earlier, you can also help manage grandparents and visitor flow.

Keep in mind that some have a hard time connecting with the baby at this stage. Some parents need a more interactive experience with the infant to bond, and newborns do not return smiles just yet. Babies do, however, already know the sound of their parents' voices; they've been hearing it in utero for months, so they already recognize you even if they can't give the visual signals yet. And every moment spent with your baby is going to help that first smile come sooner.

Q. It feels so strange to be back at work when I know my newborn is at home. What can I do to help feel more connected?

A. Many fathers feel a sense of helplessness when they have to return to work after such a short time of bonding with their new baby. But there are ways (of course this depends on your job) in which you can stay connected. Make a few calls home throughout the day and see how everyone is doing, or send a text or e-mail to let your family know you're thinking of them. When you do return home, drop everything and take the baby for a while so that Mom can get a few things done for herself. Doing what you can to reach out will help you feel more involved and connected.

Q. How can I bond with my baby when she really only sleeps and breastfeeds?

A. Reading is one of the best ways to bond with your child, and it's never too early to start. Hold her close and read a few board books, or classic poems, and at this point, there's no reason you can't simply read your baby the newspaper or the novel you've been trying to get through. She'll love the rhythmic—and familiar—sound of your voice and you'll both cherish reading together for a long time to come.

Another great way to bond with your baby right from the start is to "wear" your baby in a sling or carrier (one that fits your baby's size safely). She will get used to and be comforted by the sound of your heart, your scent, and the rhythm of your movement.

Finally, change your baby's diapers, get her dressed, and bathe her—all of these seemingly little things add up to significant interaction with your little one.

Suggested Daily Routines

Setting up a daily routine works wonders to bring much-needed structure to life with a newborn. In this section I've included some sample routines that you can try to follow in an effort to make life more manageable in these first four weeks. Each schedule varies slightly according to how you feed your baby (bottle or breast.) You don't have to follow them exactly—and of course if your baby is colicky you may drastically need to adjust—but keeping to a flexible schedule will help you adjust to life together more quickly and will help provide a supportive structure for everyone to rest and recover.

The key for this first month is to try to keep your baby on a very simple routine: Sleep, wake, play, check diaper, and feed, in that order if possible. And keep in mind that your baby may sleep more than outlined here, since it is not uncommon for babies to be awake only 10 percent of the day at this stage. During the first few weeks your baby will not be doing much playing—she will be mostly sleeping and eating. She will have a few wakeful periods during the day and this is when you can "play," and remember that play at this stage is very simple: Let your baby study your face and listen to your voice for a few minutes. When she starts to fuss, this is a sign that she has had enough. Don't try to overstimulate your baby. Toward the end of the first month, your baby will have a few more periods of wakefulness during the day.

Sample Routine for Breastfeeding Mom in Weeks 1 to 4

These routines are based on the rule that a breastfed baby needs to eat approximately nine to twelve times in a twenty-four-hour period.

TIME	TASK	SUGGESTIONS
5:00 AM	Change/ Breastfeed	Change your baby's diaper before the feed so that she's wide awake and gets the food she needs. Burp lightly after feeding.
5:40 AM	Sleep	Swaddle your baby and put her back down to sleep. It's best if you try to get back to sleep, too!
7:30 AM	Change/Play	When your baby wakes up, do not rush to feed her. Instead sing and talk to her while you change her diaper.
8:00 AM	Breastfeed	Grab a tall glass of water and make yourself comfortable either in bed or on the couch. Breastfeed your baby, then burp her.
8:40 AM	Sleep	Swaddle your baby and put her back down to sleep.
9:00 AM	Eat breakfast	Take advantage of the time you have while your baby sleeps and eat a healthy breakfast that includes protein—you'll need it to keep your energy up.
9:15 AM	Shower	It'll feel great for you to shower early. If your baby happens to be awake, simply put the bouncy seat on the floor of the bathroom and secure your baby in it.
10:00 AM	Change/Play	Hold, cuddle, and sing to your baby. Give a sponge bath to freshen her up and get her dressed. Try tummy time for a few minutes while getting down on the floor with her and talking expressively.

TIME	TASK	SUGGESTIONS
10:30 AM	Breastfeed/Play	Grab another glass of water (try to drink water during every breastfeeding session to make sure you're staying hydrated). Get cozy on the sofa or in a rocker and breastfeed your baby. Burp her and then spend a few minutes cuddling or reading a book.
11:30 AM	Change/Sleep	Continue to play and sing as you change your baby's diaper. Then swaddle her, rock to soothe her, and lay her down to sleep.
11:45 AM	Eat lunch	Again, eat something nutritious for your breastfeeding body including protein, veggies, and fresh fruit.
12:00 PM	Downtime	If you're tired, take this time to nap. If you feel up to it, get something easy started for dinner, such as chopping vegetables for a salad.
1:00 PM	Change/Breastfeed	Change your baby's diaper and sing to her while you do. Then settle into your "nest" with your water and breastfeed your baby.
1:40 PM	Walk/Play	Take a walk with your baby in the stroller or baby carrier. She'll love the fresh air and looking around at all the new surroundings—and moving around is great for you, too!
3:30 PM	Change/Breastfeed	Change your baby and describe what you're doing as you do. Grab a snack and a glass of water and settle down on the sofa to breastfeed.

TIME	TASK	SUGGESTIONS
4:15 PM	Sleep	Swaddle your baby and put her down to sleep. This is a good time of day to receive guests, because someone coming now can either bring you dinner or pick up whatever you need at the grocery store.
5:30 PM	Play	If Dad is home by this time, start prepping dinner while he plays on the floor with your baby (tummy time or reading a book).
6:30 PM	Change/ Breastfeed	Have Dad change your baby's diaper and interact while doing so. Then settle down to breastfeed.
7:00 PM	Sleep	Swaddle your baby and lay her down to sleep.
7:15 PM	Dinner	Eat a well-balanced dinner (for example, fish with rice and a side salad or steak with broccoli and potatoes will give you the nutrients to stay on track).
8:00 PM	Downtime	This is a good time to get some sleep, but if that's not possible it's also a good time to catch up on anything you've been meaning or wanting to do baby-free!
9:00 PM	Change/ Breastfeed	Talk softly to your baby as you change her. Then bring her into bed with you (or on the sofa) and breastfeed.

TIME	TASK	SUGGESTIONS
9:40 PM	Sleep	Read your baby a story and rock her. Then swaddle her and lay her back down to sleep.
12:00 AM	Change/ Breastfeed	Last feeding before a (hopefully) long stretch of sleep. If the baby wakes during the night, try to comfort her with a finger or pacifier to suck on. (Try to delay use of the pacifier for a few weeks, but if your baby isn't settling, give it a try.) Try not to stimulate her by getting her out of bed. The goal is for her to go back to sleep without another feed. Do feed her if she's upset, however.
4:30 AM	Change/ Breastfeed	Bring baby into your bed to breastfeed. Burp, change if necessary, swaddle, and return your baby to her crib. Get some sleep until the next feeding, after which you can start your day.

Sample Routine for Bottle-Feeding Mom and Dad in Weeks 1 to 4

TIME	TASK	SUGGESTIONS
6:00 AM	Change/Give bottle	Change your baby's diaper before the feed so that he's wide awake and gets what he needs. Burp thoroughly after feeding to avoid gas bubbles.
6:30 AM	Sleep	Swaddle your baby and put him back down to sleep.
7:30 AM	Eat breakfast	Eat breakfast while baby sleeps (ideally something with protein, such as eggs or yogurt, whole grain toast, and some fruit). Get your baby's bottle ready.
8:30 AM	Change/Play	When your baby wakes, don't rush into the feeding; give him a few minutes to really wake up and get hungry (fifteen minutes or so). Sing him songs, read a book, and offer tummy time for a bit.
9:00 AM	Give bottle	Get comfortable on the couch with a glass of water and feed your baby. Burp thoroughly.
10:00 AM	Sleep	Swaddle your baby and put him down for a nap.
10:15 AM	Shower/Snack	It will feel great to jump in the shower and eat a nutritious snack. You may even want to take a quick nap!

TIME	TASK	SUGGESTIONS
11:30 AM	Change/Play	Hold, cuddle, and sing to your baby. Give him a sponge bath and get him dressed. Try tummy time for a few minutes.
12:00 PM	Give bottle	Make a bottle while your baby is in the bouncy seat or swing. Then settle down in your "nest" with your baby to feed him. Burp thoroughly afterward.
1:00 PM	Change/Sleep	Change your baby's diaper while talking or singing softly. Swaddle him and lay him down to sleep. He may stay awake cooing and making noises during this time. This is OK—he needs some time to try to soothe himself. If he does not eventually fall asleep on his own, pick him up, swaddle tightly, and rock a bit before putting him back down.
1:30 PM	Lunch/Downtime	Eat a healthy lunch and check a few things off your to-do list. It'll feel great!
2:45 PM	Change/Play	Talk and sing to your baby as you change him. Then put some music on and walk around or dance with him cuddled in your arms. Try a few more moments of tummy time (this will make him stronger and stronger each time you do it!).
3:00 PM	Give bottle	Make a bottle and feed to your baby. Burp thoroughly.

TIME	TASK	SUGGESTIONS
3:40 PM	Walk/Play	Take a walk with your baby in the stroller or baby carrier. She'll love the fresh air and looking around at all the new surroundings—and moving around is great for you, too!
4:30 PM	Change/Sleep	Talk softly to your baby as you change him. Swaddle and put him down for a nap. This is a good time of day to receive guests because someone can either bring you dinner or pick up whatever you need at the grocery store.
5:30 PM	Dinner	If your partner is home, have him help you prepare a light meal. Some babies are more awake during this time of day. If baby is awake then put him in a bouncy seat or swing, or carry him around in a sling if necessary.
6:00 PM	Give bottle	This is a good time to let Dad feed the baby. They'll both benefit from the bonding and you'll benefit from a little break.
6:45 PM	Change/Bath	Together, give your baby a bath and interact calmly with him. Apply lotion if needed and dress him in comfortable pajamas.
7:30 PM	Sleep	Read your baby a story and rock him. Swaddle and lay him down to sleep.

TIME	TASK	SUGGESTIONS
9:00 PM	Change/Give bottle/Sleep	Dad can change the baby's diaper while you make a bottle. He should feed the baby once again and burp thoroughly. Re-swaddle and put him back down to sleep.
9:30 PM	Downtime	This is a good time for you to get some sleep. If that's not possible, this is a good time to relax together or get some laundry done.
12:00 AM	Change/Give bottle	Change your baby quietly, if necessary, and give him a bottle. Burp him thoroughly. A good goal is to have your baby sleep for a long stretch after this feeding. If he wakes in the wee hours, try to hold off on the feed with a pacifier, another swaddle, and/or some rocking and see he goes back to sleep.
4:30 AM	Change/Give bottle	If needed, change the baby's diaper quietly and give a bottle. Burp lightly, re-swaddle, and lay him down to get more sleep before the day starts.

· 11 ·

....

Your Baby's
Second Month:
Getting the Hang of It

....

If **you are** a first-time parent, much of your time during your baby's first four weeks will be spent just learning the basics—getting used to changing a messy diaper or giving your baby a bath amid cries of protest can be quite challenging. If this isn't your first baby, much of the first month will probably be spent helping older siblings adjust to the newest member of your family and the changes that come with him. But by the end of your baby's second month, things will begin to settle down, life will become a bit more predictable for all of you, and you will feel much more comfortable handling and caring for your baby. But just because you'll have a handle on something resembling a routine doesn't mean you won't feel like a zombie some days.

It's normal for the excitement of the first month to wear off as things become more "normal," especially if your partner returns to work. Taking care of your baby from sunup to sundown can leave you completely exhausted, and you may feel that your life has changed drastically while your partner has simply gone back to his routines. Fortunately, during this time the excitement will continue—in a different way. Your baby will begin to respond to you—he will start to smile and/or his face will light up when he sees you. This will melt your heart, and you will realize that spending time with your baby is the best thing in the whole word.

Feeding

. . . .

Your baby's feeding habits will change as he nears two months old. While during the first month you probably worried about whether or not your baby was getting enough to eat (and were tempted to feed him every time he cried), your baby's food demands in the second month will be slightly more predictable. You will see that every cry does not necessarily mean he is hungry; in fact, this would be the perfect time to try to implement a feeding schedule. Having said that, there will, of course, be times when your baby needs to eat a little sooner than you expect—especially if you're breastfeeding—so be sure stay open and flexible with any schedule you establish at this stage.

If you're breastfeeding, things should go more smoothly by this time—your baby will be more awake and should be able to feed effectively at your breast, not to mention your milk supply will be well established. Your breastfed baby will probably be feeding approximately seven to ten times per day, a slight decrease from the first month. But because it is hard to predict exactly how much breast milk your baby is getting per feeding, don't be surprised if at times she wants to feed again after only an hour or two. You will notice your baby becoming much more patient between feeds. When she wakes up, she may actually play for ten or fifteen minutes before she demands food.

If you are formula-feeding your baby, expect to feed her approximately every three hours, but keep in mind that all babies are different and there is no one specific amount of formula that she should consume on a daily basis. A good rule of thumb is that, on average, during your baby's second month she will likely drink about three to five ounces every three to four hours.

The American Academy of Pediatrics suggests that, on average, your baby should take in about two and a half ounces of formula per day for every pound of body weight. So, for a six-week-old baby weighing ten pounds, that would be about twenty-five ounces of formula per day. Most babies of this age will take three to four ounces of formula per feeding. Some babies may need more and some less; what is important is that your baby is gaining weight steadily. Your baby's pediatrician will monitor your baby's weight at each office visit.

Q. I have a breast pump at home. When should I start to use it?

A. Normally you should give yourself a few weeks of exclusive breastfeeding before you begin pumping. Your body needs to produce the right amount of milk to feed your baby, and pumping could cause an overproduction of milk that could lead to mastitis. By the third week you will know what level of breast fullness is normal for you, and you can gradually start pumping and storing milk.

However, there are some situations when you will be encouraged to pump sooner. Your health-care provider may recommend using a breast pump if your baby is having difficulty latching on or if you are using a nipple shield. Pumping is also recommended if you deliver a premature baby and the baby has to stay in the hospital a little longer than you do. In this case, pumping your breasts will help to stimulate milk production, and the milk you express can be used to feed your baby. If you have twins, pumping early on will also help to stimulate your milk production. Otherwise, pumping too much in the first few weeks may cause you to produce too much milk—which isn't impossible to readjust but does take some time and effort.

When you do begin, pump your breasts in the morning, when your milk supply is at its highest, you will be rested, and your baby will likely be content (without a feeding). Pump either right after you feed your baby or midway through the first two morning feedings.

Some women prefer to hand-express breast milk. If you do, be sure you have learned this technique from a lactation consultant or an experienced health-care provider. If you decide to use a breast pump, do your research—ask friends what they have used and talk to a lactation consultant about the right pump for your needs.

baby care tip

When you store expressed breast milk, the fats will begin to separate after a few hours (sometimes you can see the separation right after you've pumped). This is completely normal. When you need a bottle of stored, expressed milk, warm the milk by letting the bottle or bag sit in a container of warm water, and instead of shaking the milk when you're ready to feed, swirl it around a bit to mix it—this protects the antibodies.

Q. I started expressing and storing my breast milk a few days ago and now I have a few "relief" bottles in the refrigerator. What's the best way to introduce a bottle to my two-month-old?

A. It's great that you've started to store some milk—now that your baby is in his second month, there will likely come a time you'll need to be away from him for a short period. Whether it's to go to the grocery store or get a haircut, you will feel more at ease if you know that if your baby is hungry he will be fed.

If you want your baby to take a bottle of expressed milk, introduce it between weeks three and six, after breastfeeding is well established. Most babies who have an occasional bottle will go back to the breast for feedings again without any issues.

However, some babies have a difficult time with or even refuse to suck from a bottle, which can be very frustrating for anyone attempting the feed. Always remember to try to remain calm, because your baby will sense your frustration and will very likely get upset and continue to refuse. You may even find that it's easier to have a partner, family member, or friend feed your baby this way—a lot of times babies will simply eat if they are hungry and the bottle is their only food source.

baby care tip

Bottle-feed your baby in the infant carrier car seat (inside, of course, not in a moving car) or a bouncy seat if he refuses to feed when you're holding him. Make sure he is calm, and then gently place the bottle near his lips. Don't *push* the nipple into his mouth because he will likely push it back out with his tongue. Let him get used to the feel of the nipple for a minute or so and let him draw it into his mouth on his own. If your baby uses a pacifier, you can also try using that to start with and then make a quick, smooth switch to the bottle's nipple.

Q. My exclusively breastfed baby spits up a few times each day. Why is this? Should I worry that he's not eating enough?

A. Spitting up is very common in babies—it is usually the result of an immature digestive system and can happen with bottle- or breast-fed babies. If you are breastfeeding, the spit-up may be the result of your baby getting too much milk too quickly, which can happen especially when your breasts are very full. If your baby is bottle-fed and sucks too aggressively, he may also get too much too quickly and spit part of it up.

Try to feed your baby in a more upright position. Make sure the pace of the feed is steady and he's not getting too much milk too quickly, which will cause him to spit up. Pausing to burp your baby halfway through will help. After the feeding, holding your baby upright for fifteen minutes or so will help his system to digest the milk. If the spitting up continues for more than a few days and you are concerned, make an appointment with your baby's pediatrician for an evaluation and weight check. Some babies are actually "happy spitters" and do not show signs of discomfort or irritability; others may be more sensitive to belly upsets.

baby care tip

It may seem that your baby is spitting up his entire meal, but what comes up is usually only a small amount of the feeding. When it is mixed with mucus and saliva, it may look like a larger amount than it really is. Spitting in babies usually peaks between two and four months and gradually diminishes until twelve months, by which time it is usually resolved.

Q. My baby is very fussy and gassy during the night. Could he be allergic to the formula?

A. It is not unusual for babies of this age to become fussy and gassy, but this is not usually related to the belly or the formula. Despite what you may hear about allergies, milk allergies are not common, especially if the baby's parents do not have milk allergies.

The fact that your baby seems happy for most of the day and is only fussy at night might also indicate that it is probably not the formula. Both breastfed and formula-fed babies can start to become fussy at about three weeks of age and continue for the next few months. The fussing usually peaks at about six weeks and begins to get better each week after that. Every baby is different, however. Some babies have a regular time of day (usually late afternoon) when they start to fuss; others are periodically fussy throughout the day; and some become restless and irritable at night. You may actually be more aware of your baby's behavior at night because the house is quieter then and you are probably trying to go to sleep. Try your best to stay calm and soothe your baby (soothing and sleeping tips will be discussed later in this chapter). However, if you think your baby's discomfort is related to your formula, take him to his pediatrician for an evaluation.

Q. **My breastfed baby has been very irritable lately, and this morning when I changed his diaper I noticed blood in his stool. What does this mean?**

A. Your baby is probably not allergic to your breast milk but rather to something in your diet such as dairy products. Cow's milk products are the most common cause of food allergies in babies, although soy, wheat, corn, eggs, and peanuts have also been known to affect certain babies. Symptoms that your baby is allergic to something in your breast milk include bloody mucus in the stools, body rash, hives, eczema, fussiness, and irritability. If you suspect your baby is allergic to a particular food, eliminate that food from your diet for two to three weeks and see if his symptoms improve. Two weeks may seem like a long time, but cow's milk protein can remain in your breast milk for one to two weeks, and then it will take another week or two for the protein to get out of the baby's body. Generally you can expect your baby's symptoms to start improving within five to seven days from when you first eliminated the offending food.

Q. **My husband is lactose-intolerant and my breastfed baby seems to be reacting when I consume dairy products. Could my breastfed baby be lactose-intolerant as well? Should I stop eating dairy?**

A. Your baby may be sensitive to dairy products, but it is highly unlikely he is lactose-intolerant. If your baby is sensitive to the dairy in your diet, he is sensitive to the cow's milk proteins, not lactose, that pass into breast milk, so it will not help to switch to lactose-free products. If you think that your baby is sensitive to dairy, you must omit these foods from your diet. If you are formula-feeding your baby, your pediatrician may recommend switching to soy or a hypoallergenic or hydrolyzed formula. A hypoallergenic formula contains broken-down proteins, which are less likely to trigger an allergic reaction.

It is also possible that your baby is not sensitive to dairy or lactose at all but instead just reacting to the acidity of some of the foods you're eating. Try to monitor what you eat and how your baby reacts to see which foods you might want to omit.

baby care tip

When you are trying to avoid dairy products because your baby is sensitive to milk protein, milk is obviously not the only food to avoid. Here are some common foods that contain this protein: artificial butter flavor, butter, buttermilk, casein, cheese, chocolate, cottage cheese, cream, custard, goat's milk, goat cheese, kefir, lactalbumin, lactose, milk, nougat, pudding, sour cream, whey, and yogurt. Kosher foods marked "Pareve" are dairy-free.

Q. My breastfed baby still has several loose bowel movements per day. Is this normal or is it my milk? Do I still have to keep track of his pooping patterns?

A. You must be feeding him well, since what goes in must come out! Yes, frequent loose stools are normal since your baby's digestive system is not yet completely mature. Expect his bowel habits to be irregular for at least a few more weeks. Eventually your baby will have a bowel movement once or twice per day, for the most part. And you no longer have to keep track of the number of bowel movements—it sounds like he's pretty regular at this point!

Q. My breastfed baby has not had a bowel movement in a few days. He does not seem unhappy or uncomfortable, but he normally has dirty diapers several times a day. Is he constipated?

A. As long as your baby is having soft bowel movements, it is unlikely that your baby is constipated. It's just that his digestive system is starting to work better, and when that happens the frequency of his stools will decrease (most often to once or twice a day). But you want to make sure that when your baby does pass a stool, the consistency is soft, not hard or pellet-shaped. If you are concerned because your baby has not recently had a bowel movement, call your pediatrician.

Sleeping

Your baby's second month allows for more sleeping options in both sleeping arrangements and sleeping routines. During her first month, your baby learns that she can trust her parents because she will be attended to whenever she cries, including times you think she "should" be sleeping. This part of normal psychological infant development should be fairly established in month two, which makes it a more appropriate time to regulate the times your baby sleeps.

Trying to establish a sleep routine for your baby may be particularly helpful if you yourself feel utterly sleep-deprived, as one mom I worked with did. She called and told me that she hadn't slept in weeks because her eight-week-old baby would only sleep while on her. Whenever she put the baby down, he would sleep for about fifteen minutes and then wake up. Realizing that the family just needed a little help starting and sticking to an effective sleep routine, I spent a couple days with them recommending some strategies (which I will share in this section). Within three days this ecstatic mom called me with good news: The whole family had gotten some sleep! She checked back two weeks later and, although the baby did have a few setbacks, the overall sleep situation had improved drastically—making for a very happy family all around.

Sleeping Arrangements

Times have really changed when it comes to babies and sleeping arrangements, and it all comes down to safety. Although different families will have different philosophies, it is important to seriously consider the AAP recommendations of keeping baby in your room but in a *separate* bed for the first six months—ideally a year. Cosleeping used to be considered disruptive to an infant's sleep as well as parents', but as long as you establish a consistent routine, everyone should sleep well and, more importantly, *safely*.

Sleeping Routines

Like the sleeping arrangements, your baby's bedtime routine—or absence of one—will also depend on your own goals for sleep. If you are interested in establishing a sleep routine for your baby, then you should dedicate some time *and patience* to it during month two. Your baby may fuss a bit at first when you put him to bed and leave the room, but eventually he will learn to fall asleep on his own—which is a great sleeping habit to adapt so early. This is not the "crying it out" method—there is a big difference between a distressed crying baby and a whimpering sleepy baby.

Your baby needs between fifteen and sixteen hours of sleep in a twenty-four-hour period. Most babies do not sleep through the night at this point, so your first goal should be to get a five-hour stretch. Establish a bedtime sometime between 8 PM and 11 PM. He'll probably wake once or twice during the night to feed, but these sleep periods will start to get a bit longer during this month. If you want your baby to take more regular naps, observe the times your baby tends to get sleepy during the day and create the nap schedule around that.

Q. I put my baby down this evening at eight and he started to fuss right away. When I picked him up, he quieted down. I rocked him to sleep within five minutes and put him into his crib, and within another five minutes he was up and starting to fuss. What am I doing wrong?

A. Let's think about what is happening. It is your baby's bedtime and he is obviously tired, since when you rocked him he fell back asleep in five minutes. Don't confuse your baby's "fussing" for cries of distress.

Your baby's fussing really means, "Mom, I'm trying to figure out how to fall asleep on my own. I've never done this before and I'm trying to figure out how it all works." Let him fuss for a while and then walk out of the room. If he starts to get upset, give him a few minutes and then go back in and calm him down without getting him out of the crib. Rub his tummy gently, let him suck on a pacifier, and tell him that you love him but that it is time for him to go to bed. When he calms, walk out of the room and give him another five minutes. Repeat the process of calming him. By not picking him up, you are helping him learn how to fall asleep on his own. Continue this routine for daytime naps, too, for a week and you will be amazed how quickly your baby will learn to fall asleep on his own. It takes some effort and discipline but there are benefits—helping him to learn a great skill and hopefully getting some sleep or extra downtime for yourself!

Q. My baby falls asleep after I feed him at night and usually has a good three- to five-hour stretch, but then he is awake on and off from about midnight. I'm exhausted. Why won't my baby sleep?

A. Your baby will sleep once he learns to fall asleep on his own. Instead of putting your baby down to sleep immediately after he eats, when he's really sleepy, try to put him down for the night still a bit awake so he can learn to get himself to sleep. It sounds like he is associating sleep with being fed, so as long as you continue he will have a hard time learning to stay asleep for the rest of the night. Instead, establish a bedtime routine: Feed him a little earlier than you normally do to make sure he stays alert, and then read a story for a few minutes before putting him down.

We all wake up several times during the night, but we are able to get back to sleep—and most of the time we don't even realize or remember we were awake. Your baby, too, will wake up several times each night and needs to learn how to go back to sleep without being fed, held, or rocked in your arms. It's OK if your baby fusses and even cries a bit. As I mentioned, you can always go calm him down. Your baby may need to cry a bit to figure it out, and this won't be easy for you—especially if it's 2 AM and all you want to do is go to sleep. Of course, it is easier to pick up your baby and rock him until he falls asleep so you can get back to bed, but understand that this routine will continue to happen night after night. Next time your baby starts to fuss in the middle of the night, wait a few minutes before you respond. He may actually be able to fall back asleep on his own.

> ### baby care tip
> When your baby needs to sleep yet cries when you put him down, try to let him settle himself for a few minutes before going back into the room. Most babies will take ten or fifteen minutes to settle themselves and then fall asleep for a nap. If your baby is crying frantically then pick him up, re-swaddle, rock for a few minutes to calm him down, and put him back in the crib.

Soothing

Many babies of this age will begin to have periods of fussiness throughout the day. As mentioned earlier, this is normal and is seen in both breast- and bottle-fed babies. This fussiness will likely continue over the next few weeks and peak at about week six. After that your baby's fussy periods will begin to ease, and may be gone or at least greatly diminish by the end of month three. Some babies are fussier than others, and if your little one does fuss a lot, those early weeks of bliss with your newborn can quickly turn into days of feeling like you're at the end of your rope.

Colic

I'm sure you've heard the word *colic*—about 20 to 25 percent of babies will have periods of colic (long periods of extreme fussiness for no apparent reason) during these early months of the fourth trimester. Over the years much research has been done on colic, but the exact cause of why a baby constantly cries is unknown. Colic comes from a Greek word, *kolikos*, which means colon, which is why for years it's been thought to be an intestinal problem. Experts blame it on immature digestive systems, immature nervous systems, allergies, hypersensitivities, or even maternal anxiety. These are still all theories and many experts still do not agree about the cause of this condition. One thing is for certain—it is absolutely not Mom's fault. Read on to learn more about whether or not your baby may be colicky and what you can do to soothe him.

Q. My baby is six weeks old and has suddenly started to cry for several hours late in the day. She is not hungry and her diaper is clean—she should be relatively happy but she just keeps crying. How do I know if my baby has colic?

A. Many pediatricians and baby experts use the rule of threes: If your baby is less than three months old, cries for three or more hours at a time, and cries for three or more days per week, she has colic. Take your baby to her pediatrician to rule out any medical issue that could be making her cry, and if she has a clean bill of health, practice the soothing techniques explained in chapter 10 to get you through the next few weeks. Most babies will outgrow this behavior by three months.

baby care tip

To survive colic, make sure you get a one- or two-hour break every day if you can. Talk to your friends and family members and try to set up a schedule where someone will come over for a few hours each day so you can get away from the crying—even if it is just for an hour. Remember that crying will always sound worse to your ears than to anyone else's. Your family members will likely be happy to help out and care for your baby so you can take a much-needed rest. Constant crying can make any parent feel angry and even resentful—this is normal when you are faced with a baby who is crying for hours.

Keep reminding yourself that colic has nothing to do with you, and that it will eventually pass and fade into distant memory. However, if none of your soothing efforts work, it is important that you periodically put your baby down in a safe place (like a crib) and take a five- or ten-minute break. She will be just fine and it's best for *both* of you! Sit down, have a cup of tea, or even get a few minutes of fresh air to help ease the feelings of frustration. Always ask for help if you have thoughts or feelings about harming your baby; and keep in mind that most mothers have unsettling thoughts at some point. Having them does not make you a bad mother.

When It's Not Colic

If this is your first baby, trying to figure out if your baby is sick, has colic, or has something else can be difficult. Knowing what to do and how to soothe your baby when he is sick can be tricky, too. While the chances of your baby becoming sick at two months (or really anytime in the newborn stage) are slim, it's good to know the signs and have a plan in place should it happen. Here are some signs that your baby might be coming down with something:

Appearance—Is your baby pale? Does he have an unusual rash on his body or his face?

Behavior—Is your baby acting differently? (By this time you should be able to spot a difference in behavior.) Is she uninterested in playing? Is she crying more than usual? Is she crying at times of the day when she is usually happy? Is she sleeping more than usual?

Feeding—Is he feeding less? Is he uninterested in breastfeeding, or pushing the bottle away?

Breathing—Does she have a cough or a stuffy nose?

Fever—Does he feel unusually sweaty? Does he have a fever?

If your baby has one or more of these symptoms, she very well may be sick. Call your baby's pediatrician and explain what's going on. They will tell you whether or not to bring your baby in for an evaluation. Do not give your baby any medication at home before talking to your pediatrician first. But trust your inner wisdom—no one knows your baby like you do. If you think something is not right, then go with your instincts.

baby care tip

If your baby feels warm but does not have any of the above symptoms, he is probably not sick. Undress him or take a layer of clothing off and see if he cools down. Feeding him might also help, because if your baby is thirsty or a bit dehydrated, he may appear warm. If he still feels warm after eating, place a thermometer under his arm and see if he has a fever. If he does, take a rectal temperature to make sure.

Q: How do I take my baby's temperature?

A: There are two good methods for taking your baby's temperature—under the arm and rectally. Many pediatricians prefer the rectal method since it is typically a more accurate reading of your baby's core body temperature. If you are not comfortable with taking your baby's rectal temperature, take it under the arm and ask your pediatrician to show you how to take a rectal temperature at your first baby checkup. (It's not as bad as it sounds and won't hurt your baby!)

Purchase a digital thermometer, as they tend to be the easiest to use. Do not buy one that contains mercury. Other types of thermometers such as the ear devices and sensor strips are not recommended right now and often fail to get accurate readings. You may want to buy two thermometers and mark one "A" for *arm* and the other "R" for *rectal*.

NORMAL TEMPERATURES

- **Rectal:** 99.6°F or 37.5°C
- **Arm:** 97.5°F or 36.5°C

If your baby's temperature registers above normal, contact your pediatrician immediately. Until your baby is about three to four months old, he cannot effectively fight infections because his immune system is still immature. Once you've spoken with your baby's pediatrician (or the one on call, depending on the time), you'll most likely have a care plan put in place if there's any cause for concern.

If your baby is sick and has been seen and treated medically, it may still take some time for him to get back to his "normal" happy self. Until then, cuddling and rocking your baby close, rubbing his back, and speaking softly and lovingly are the best soothing techniques—and these will come instinctively to you! While you may have to resign yourself to the fact that you probably won't sleep as much during this period as you normally do, other soothing techniques I've discussed, such as swaddling and giving your baby a pacifier, may help as well.

baby care tip

Between the ages of four and eight weeks, many babies start to sound stuffy and congested when they breathe through the nose. Our family pediatrician used the term "snurgle" eighteen years ago, when I brought my then four-week-old baby in. Over the last fifteen years I have seen hundreds of babies with the same thing and I still love using the term "snurgle"—it's a cross between a sniffle, a snort, and a gurgle. Parents often interpret this sound as a cold, but if this is the only symptom, your baby is most likely not sick. The congestion is caused by a buildup of mucus in the respiratory tract, which makes your baby's breathing sound noisy because he breathes through his nose. It is not harmful and will resolve by about eight weeks.

Q. I tried swaddling, but my baby doesn't seem to like it and cries when I'm doing it. Should I stop trying to swaddle?

A. Most babies don't like to be moved around much. Notice how your baby cries when you change his diaper. Try swaddling your baby again, and when you're done, pick him up and gently rock him back and forth in your arms. Babies also like sounds—use soft classical music, your soft humming voice, or even a white noise machine as you swaddle. You are trying to re-create your baby's feelings of being in the womb. Most babies will settle down and enjoy the swaddle. If he still does not settle, take him out of the swaddle; he may not be interested in sleeping at this point. Don't give up on the swaddle just because your baby didn't like it once or twice.

Q. Can I spoil my baby by picking her up all the time?

A. You cannot spoil your baby at this age by picking her up to soothe her. Your baby needs to know that she can depend on you to help when she is distressed. Newborns cannot learn to soothe themselves until between three and four months of age, so you will need to provide her with the comforts she needs. When she is tired and needs to sleep, try to let her settle herself for a few minutes. Most babies will take ten to fifteen minutes to settle themselves and then fall asleep for a nap. If your baby is crying frantically, then pick her up, re-swaddle, rock for a few minutes, and put her back in the crib. (I don't recommend letting her remain in a distressed state at any point, but it is OK for her to make a few grunts and fuss.) It is not until about four to six months that a baby can start to associate crying with getting picked up. So until then hold your baby as much as you like, guilt-free. They are only this young once, so take advantage of this special time with your spoil-proof newborn!

Development

When your baby is two months old, you will notice her becoming much more interested in the world around her as her senses continue to develop. What does your baby like? Your baby likes you the best! She wants to see, hear, and be touched by you. Here's a breakdown of your baby's senses at this point, and some ways you can stimulate them:

Touch

Your baby will continue to be sensitive to touch and will enjoy being held and cuddled. After bath time, a soothing touch activity can be to lightly massage mild lotion into your baby's legs, arms, back, belly, and face.

Tummy Time and Other Play

In addition to experiencing touch from you, your baby will now also benefit from exploring her own sense of touch through simple exercises. One of the best is "tummy time." (You can actually start this activity as early as one week old, for short periods throughout the day!) Engaging your baby in tummy time on a regular basis will help to strengthen the neck and head muscles necessary for crawling, walking, and other physical motor skills such as climbing.

Tummy time will also help prevent positional plagiocephaly, the so-called flat head syndrome, which can develop if your baby spends too much time on her back while she's too young to move her head on her own. Your baby will spend many hours on her back while sleeping and eating, so getting her onto her tummy for some activity when she's awake is important.

Your baby may not like tummy time at first, but don't give up. She'll get used to it, and will eventually enjoy exploring and touching her environment from that angle. Start out by laying your baby on her tummy for a few minutes at a time. If she fusses, give her a few minutes to get comfortable. You can also place a breastfeeding pillow or rolled-up blanket under her chest to help keep her head elevated. Join your baby on the floor so she can look at your face. Make tummy time a fun playtime experience—talk to her and make silly faces. As your baby gets older she'll start to imitate you, and the length of time she will tolerate tummy time will increase.

baby care tip

Babies love to look at faces, even their own. To mix up your tummy time activity, get a mirror and place it so your baby can see her face. She will have a ball looking at herself and seeing another baby in the mirror. Put on some fun music and enjoy!

If your baby develops a preference to tilt his head in one direction over another, or if he seems to have limited neck movement, he may have a condition called torticollis. Some babies are born with this condition, which is usually caused by tightness in the muscle that connects the breastbone and collarbone to the skull. This tightness usually develops because of the way the baby was positioned in the uterus during pregnancy. Don't worry—if you don't notice this, your pediatrician will during your baby's routine visits. Your pediatrician may refer you and your baby to a physical therapist or may simply teach you some simple neck exercises you can do daily with your baby. The idea is to get your baby to turn her head to the side that she normally doesn't prefer, and tummy time can really benefit a baby with torticollis because you can simply favor one side while you're playing and interacting on the floor.

baby care tip

If your baby has torticollis, lay her on her changing table with her head to the side that she doesn't prefer. Play with her in this position—show her toys and sing her a song so she gets used to moving her head in that direction.

In addition to tummy time, your baby will also begin to enjoy other types of interactive play, including:

Play gym, play mat, or bouncy seat—Lay your baby under a so-called play gym or place him in a bouncy seat and let him observe the dangling toys. In time he will begin to try to bat at the dangling objects in front of him and feel their different textures.

Rattle—If you open your baby's hand and place the small rattle in it, he is likely to grasp and hold on to it. Remember to use a rattle that has a low "bonk" factor, because although your baby's movements will be less jerky at this point, he will probably move his hands toward his face. A soft rattle will not hurt him if he hits himself unexpectedly.

Music—Listen to music and sing songs that require physical interaction. This can mean simply dancing with your baby so he can feel the rhythm of your movement, or it can mean helping your baby clap, tap, or roll her arms along!

Hearing

Also continuing to develop is your baby's sense of hearing. Not only will your baby still be attuned to the sound of your voice but she will also enjoy—and be curious about—listening to the sounds in the world around her. While it's important for your baby to have some quiet time for awake periods during the day, go ahead and fill the rest of it with various sounds. His brain will absorb it all and develop accordingly.

Learn a few baby tunes and sing them to him several times a day, perhaps during routine events such as diaper changes or feedings. While you play your baby can be on your lap, lying in a bouncy seat, or on the floor. Before long, you'll hear your baby's first outright belly laugh!

baby care tip

Make up songs using the tunes of nursery rhyme songs you are familiar with. For example, when my daughter was a baby I used "Twinkle, twinkle, little star" to sing, "Mommy loves you, yes, I do / Mommy loves you, yes, I do." I always just made up my own songs using the tunes of songs that I knew. The words made no sense and didn't rhyme but my baby had no idea; she just loved hearing my voice, and I loved watching her face light up when I sang to her. You can even simply describing what you're doing, like changing a diaper or putting the dishes away.

Sight

Your baby can now see much farther than she could when she was first born—almost three feet. Familiar faces, especially yours, will light up her world. Your interaction with her should include lots of face-to-face time and eye contact.

At this age your baby will continue to prefer toys, books, and mobiles that have contrasting and bright colors. It won't be until seven months or so that your baby will be interested in lighter color combinations.

baby care tip

Buy some board books (baby books with thick cardboard pages) so that when your baby looks away or becomes uninterested, you can tap on the book to get her attention again. Choose books that have simple, large graphics. Your baby will prefer these to books with lots of small images on the page.

Taste and Smell

Your baby has a very sharp, tuned-in sense of taste and smell. Your baby is used to your scent and is soothed and comforted by it. In utero, he got used to tasting your diet through the amniotic fluid, and if you are breastfeeding, your baby continues to be exposed to the foods you eat through your breast milk. Babies are born with a sweet tooth and will generally gulp down breast milk or formula because they are both sweet. Even if you have been exclusively breastfeeding, at this point your baby is not likely to have any problems drinking formula.

Another way to engage your baby's sense of smell is to have him sit in a bouncy seat or swing (in a safe spot) in the kitchen while you cook meals. He'll enjoy the wide variety of scents.

Milestones

· · · · · · · · · · · · ·

Q. My baby smiles in her sleep. When will she smile at me?

A. The first smiles you see on your baby will probably be when she is sleeping, or you may assume they're just gas. Sometime between six and eight weeks (or sometimes even later), you will see your baby smile back at you. Instead of communicating only through crying, your baby will start to become more social this month and begin smiling for real. Those first smiles are usually reserved for Mom, Dad, and familiar people in your baby's life. Expect your baby to continue to expand her smiling skills, and in a few months she will be smiling at the world.

At the end of the second month your baby may:

- Hold her head up steadily
- Try to roll over in one direction
- Raise her chest when lying on her stomach for tummy time
- Smile
- Respond to loud sounds
- Begin to make noises and cooing sounds
- Focus on a wide variety of objects

At your baby's two-month pediatrician appointment, your baby's health-care provider will:

- Perform a complete physical exam
- Measure your baby's height, weight, and head circumference
- Assess your baby's growth and development
- Begin immunizations according to the recommended schedule

Mom in Month Two

. . . .

Q. I am constantly criticizing my husband about how he takes care of our baby. What is wrong with me?

A. Unfortunately, this is a normal reaction to the demands of post-partum life. Your hormones and extreme sleep deprivation, bundled with the recovery from the major physical feat of birth, can add up to a potentially grumpy persona. Do yourself and your family a favor and make sleep a priority! When you do find yourself getting worked up, take a few deep breaths and count to ten before reacting or criticizing.

It could also just be your maternal instinct to want to be in control of every aspect of your baby's care. But it is important to remember that taking care of your baby is a learning experience for both of you. Making an effort to communicate in a positive way from the very beginning will benefit your family now and in the future.

Q. Now that I'm alone with the baby all day, I find that at 4 PM I am still in my pajamas, I haven't showered, and the house is a mess. Why can't I manage this?

A. Legions of women before you have wandered through the day in their pajamas, often covered in spit-up. This will happen on occasion, no doubt, but turn to the last pages of this chapter and read the suggested daily routines. They will give you some ideas on how to go about structuring your day, including getting yourself out of the house for a short time each day (essential for your physical and mental well-being) and making yourself feel like you are part of the world at large again. With regard to the housework, cut yourself some slack. You'll get to that; just take care of yourself first. And don't forget, you can always put your baby in a bouncy seat or any other safe spot to play in the bathroom while you take a shower—it may not be ideal for you, but you'll feel a lot better!

Q. Sometimes I am so overwhelmed that I have unsettling thoughts about my baby. I feel guilty. Am I a bad mom?

A. All new moms and dads feel overwhelmed—it's normal. This is all new for you. Before the baby, you had only yourself to worry about, but now you have a little one who is totally dependent on you. The good news is that at this stage all your baby really wants is food, sleep, play, and hugs. Nothing else.

No, you're not a bad mother and there's no need to feel guilty, either. The only time new moms (including you, I'll bet) really have a few minutes to themselves is when the baby naps, and newborns often only nap for fifteen to twenty minutes before they start to stir and fuss. You may feel an enormous amount of pressure to accomplish something in that short period, but it's important to realize—and accept—that for the first few months that may not be realistic. Just taking a shower and getting dressed takes a lot of time and cooperation from your baby, and there may be days when she is fussy and just cannot settle herself. On days like that, even the "best" mothers have anxious thoughts. If this happens, just put your baby in her bed and take a breather. Sometimes you just have to ignore the crying for five minutes. Your baby will be all right.

As I discussed in chapter 10, if the feeling of being overwhelmed does not go away and you are feeling detached from your baby, this may be a sign that you are suffering from postpartum depression. Not wanting to be around the baby is a sign that you may need professional help. Call your health-care provider with any concerns you may have.

Q. Lately my husband and I have been bickering over everything. I'm beginning to resent the fact that it seems like his life has not really changed as much as mine has. He gets up every morning, goes to the gym, and then goes to work, and only comes home at 6 PM I'm lucky even to get a shower these days. What is happening to me?

A. What you are feeling is a common topic of discussion among most new moms. If you are in a weekly playgroup, you are likely to hear that other moms feel the same way about their partners. Your lives as a couple have changed significantly, so remember to keep the lines of communication open no matter how stressed or upset you feel. Talking about things can make you feel better and help to resolve the situation without leaving lingering resentment. Tell your partner what exactly is bothering you, and really listen and try to understand where he is coming from as well. This is new territory for both of you and you'll have a happier family if everyone feels heard, understood, and respected as you learn and grow through this stage.

baby care tip

Join a weekly play group! There's nothing better than being able to talk to other parents who are going through (or have gone through) exactly what you're experiencing. Sharing the joys, and perhaps the stresses, of parenthood can really help you put things in perspective and not feel so alone. And, of course, it's a great opportunity for your baby to play among her peers!

Exercise

As you come up on six weeks postpartum, you will likely have clearance from your health-care provider to start exercising again. Regardless of how active you were before you got pregnant, at this point your body is still getting acclimated to its post-pregnancy state, so it's important to start off slow and gradually increase your workouts. If you weren't all that active before, this is the perfect time to start making exercise a part of your life. It will not only increase your overall health but will make you look and feel great.

Enrolling in a parent/baby exercise or yoga class is one of the best ways to get in shape because such classes offer a great workout, you can bring your baby along, and you can socialize with other parents (which can be particularly helpful in the winter, when you may feel cooped up and perhaps a little isolated). Keep in mind that these classes tend to be designed for moms and their babies, but it never hurts to inquire about whether dads/partners can enroll as well. Some established programs are Stroller Strides, Baby Boot Camp, and StrollerFit, but you may find plenty of other options in your area, including at a local physical therapy clinic.

Many parents I've worked with over the years have mentioned that they really want to start exercising but just don't have the time or the money for a gym membership or structured class. But there are actually dozens of other ways to get fit at little to no cost when the time is right for you. Here are a few ideas:

Walk—Make it a priority to get out for a walk at least once a day, ideally for at least thirty minutes. This is a perfect way to get exercise and fresh air, which, as you'll see, can make a world of difference to your body and mind. You can switch things up by going for a little hike in the woods with your baby in a carrier one day and a walk around the neighborhood in the stroller the next.

Dance—One great way to bond with your two-month-old while getting your heart pumping is to put on some music and dance! You can gently sway your baby back and forth to the music while holding him, or settle him in a breastfeeding pillow and do more exaggerated, quick-paced moves, which he will no doubt happily watch!

Get an exercise DVD—Search for an exercise, dance, or yoga DVD or online video that suits your exercise goals. There are literally hundreds to choose from and they can cost as little as eight dollars. Be sure to check customer reviews of each DVD, as they can really give you a good idea if it's the right one for you. Once you've gotten one you like, pop that DVD in once the baby is down for a nap (or she may actually enjoy watching you from her bouncy seat or right there on the floor!).

The climate when you hit your six weeks postpartum date may dictate what kind of exercise, if any, you engage in at first. But whether it's the dead of winter with weekly snowstorms and below-freezing temperatures, a hundred-degree summer, or a rainy and cold spring, there are many ways—including braving the weather—to get your body moving again. Of course, if it really is too cold or too warm to be out with your baby, go with your indoor exercise options (just talk to your baby's pediatrician about high-risk weather conditions). Remember, "getting your body back" won't just happen overnight—the key is to set long-term health goals and just keep moving.

Checking in with Dad (or Partner)

· · · · · · · · · · · ·

Very few parents feel romantic toward each other in the weeks following childbirth, for some pretty understandable reasons. It's important to remember, however, that being a new parent doesn't mean you're no longer a sexual being. Even if you don't have the time, stamina, or interest in having sexual intercourse, you and your partner can still find ways to express your love for each other.

baby care tips

Dads and partners: When you and your partner do start to resume sex, be sure to discuss your birth control options. Many people are under the false assumption that it's not possible to get pregnant while breastfeeding, but it certainly is! If you don't want another baby just yet, decide upon a method that works best for you and use it. Your partner can always get recommendations and prescriptions from her health-care provider.

Love through talk—Keep the lines of communication open no matter how stressed you feel. Remember that you're both going through huge life changes. Talking about them can help you feel closer. Frame complaints so that they don't sound accusatory: Instead of saying, "You shouldn't ___," for example, try, "I feel ___ when you ___."

Love through laughter—When your life has turned upside-down and you've never felt so exhausted, it's as appropriate to laugh about it as to cry. Poke fun at your own mistakes and situation together.

Love through escape—Leave your baby in the care of a trusted relative or sitter while you go on a date. See a movie, go out for dinner or dessert, or do something else you can enjoy together. Just being away for a couple of hours can recharge you.

Love through touching—Sex isn't all about intercourse. Kissing, cuddling, caressing, and other kinds of physical intimacy don't require a lot of energy and can help you relax.

Love through time—Remember that these topsy-turvy weeks are temporary.

baby care tip

Take photos and record videos of your little one even if he doesn't "do" much, because in just a month or two, you won't believe the immense changes. You'll feel so proud at how far your little one has come!

Suggested Daily Routines

Many parents return to work in the second month, commonly after six weeks. If you are bottle-feeding, plan to use seven to nine bottles a day, each containing three to six ounces of expressed breast milk or formula. If you are breastfeeding, your baby may need to feed at the breast nine to twelve times a day.

Sample Routine for Two Working Parents of Bottle-Fed Eight-Week-Old Baby

TIME	TASK	SUGGESTIONS
5:45 AM	Change/Give bottle	Change your baby's diaper before the feed so that she's wide awake and gets what she needs. Burp thoroughly after feeding.
6:30 AM	Bath	Baby gets a "sponge bath" to remove any formula or spit-up that may have run into the folds of her neck overnight. Baby gets dressed for the day.
6:45 AM	Play/Family gets ready	Put baby on her stomach for some brief "tummy time" and a back rub. Take turns showering, getting ready, and eating breakfast.

TIME	TASK	SUGGESTIONS
7:30 AM	Leave for child care/ Child-care provider arrives	Either pack up the car with essentials for the day at child care, or, if you have someone come to your home have your child-care provider come a little before you leave for work so you can give them an update and instructions.
8:00 AM	Dropoff/Leave for work	Drop your baby off with the child-care provider and leave for work.
8:00 AM – 5:30 PM	Child care	The child-care provider feeds and takes care of your baby according to your recommendations. You receive a report of your baby's day when you pick her up. She will drink three or so bottles during the day.
6:00 PM	Play/Give bottle	Hold, cuddle, and sing to your baby. Give her a bottle and burp thoroughly.
6:45 PM	Change/Sleep	Gently talk and sing to your baby, then swaddle and put her down to sleep.
7:00 PM	Dinner/Downtime	Enjoy a healthy meal and catch up on the to-do list. Get things ready and packed for the morning.
8:30 PM	Change/Bath	Give baby a sponge bath and get her dressed. Try tummy time for a few minutes.
9:00 PM	Give bottle	Make a bottle and let Dad/Partner feed and bond with the baby. Burp thoroughly.

TIME	TASK	SUGGESTIONS
9:45 PM	Sleep	Swaddle and rock your baby, then put her down to sleep.
11:15 PM	Give bottle	Baby drinks a bottle called a "dream feed": Feed the baby, but try to keep things as quiet and still as possible. This will help to stretch everyone's sleep as long as possible during the night.
4:15 AM–6:00 AM	Change/Give bottle	Baby may stir, but when left alone could go back to sleep within about fifteen minutes. Once it's really time to eat, change the baby first and then give the bottle.

As with the first month of your baby's life, the second month will bring new challenges and pleasures. While you'll still be grappling for some semblance of a routine for your baby and will likely remain somewhat sleep-deprived, your baby will be growing every day with each cuddle, smile, and song you provide. Whether you feel bittersweet about your baby's rapid growth or look forward to leaving the newborn phase behind, just keep breathing and enjoying this time. Although each month will bring a new set of challenges, you'll continue to settle into your role as Mom, which will make everything a little easier, more predictable, and even *more* fun!

· 12 ·

Your Baby's Third Month:
The Newborn Homestretch

As your baby nears the three month mark, you will find yourself looking back on what an exciting adventure your first months of parenthood have been. At this point, your new baby will not exactly be a newborn anymore, as so many changes will have taken place in such a short amount of time. Things will finally be falling into place and life will take on a new familiar routine. You will no longer feel clumsy handling your baby; in fact, you can probably change a diaper and talk on the phone at the same time! And if there are other siblings in the home, your baby will likely be a completely integrated family member. She may now recognize family members, smile at familiar faces, even talk in her own baby language. This is only the beginning; as your baby continues to grow and develop, her distinct personality will begin to emerge—and you will love every second of it!

Of course, along with the return to relative normalcy that comes with having a three-month-old baby—versus a one- or two-month-old newborn—you should be aware of a few transitions. If you are returning to work, for example, you may feel anxious about how you and your baby will handle the change. Once you spend nine months pregnant and the following several weeks in the constant company of your baby, it's hard to imagine being separated even for a few hours. This chapter will address some of the concerns parents have when they return to work, and will offer tips and solutions to help ease the transition for everyone.

Another important shift to be aware of as your baby turns three months old is in development and the level of your interaction together. You will want to spend more time stimulating your baby's development—which primarily occurs through language—and this chapter will give you suggestions on how to best to do that.

Although you will likely feel settled into your baby's sleeping and eating routines at this point, I will also address some common questions about feeding, soothing, sleeping patterns, and the quality of life for Mom and Dad.

Feeding

At this stage of your baby's development, breast milk and formula are still your only feeding options. Solid foods are off limits for at least another one to three months because your baby's digestive system is still developing. You may be breastfeeding, bottle-feeding, or a combination of both to feed your baby, and he's old enough to decide when he's hungry—and he'll very likely tell you in his own way! Learn to read your baby's cues that he wants to eat and try to stick to a flexible feeding schedule that works well for both you and baby. Your baby will stop eating when he is full, and as long as his weight gain has stayed within normal limits for the first three months there is no reason to push or force him to eat more. Your baby will be hungrier some days than others; don't expect him to eat for the same length of time during every feed. Your baby will be hungrier when his body is undergoing a growth spurt (typically growth spurts occur two weeks after birth, at six weeks, at three months, and at six months), and if he is not feeling well he may want less food. Also remember that because your baby is a little older, it is not necessary to respond to his every whimper with a breast or a bottle. If you have recently fed him and he is fussing, he may be trying to tell you that he needs his diaper changed, wants to be played with, or needs to nap.

At three months of age babies breastfeed about six to eight times per day. The length of the feeding is determined by factors such as how aggressive a feeder your baby is and how full your breasts are with milk. Some breastfed babies are completely satisfied after eating for twenty minutes from only one breast, while others take a little longer to feed and may want to nurse from both breasts.

The amount of formula your three-month-old baby takes depends on his weight. A three-month-old baby weighs between nine and sixteen pounds, with an average weight of thirteen. Based on our formula calculation from chapter 11, a thirteen-pound baby will take approximately thirty-two ounces per day. Until your baby takes solid foods, multiply the baby's weight by two to three ounces to get the approximate number of ounces of formula your baby needs. Babies should not exceed thirty-two to thirty-three ounces of formula per day. Most will have approximately six five-ounce bottles per day.

Knowing this basic information is helpful but remember that babies eat when they are hungry and stop when they are full. Your baby's appetite will vary from day to day— that's why it is important to read your baby's cues. If he is refusing his bottle and you think it is time to eat, he may be telling you he is tired and needs a quick nap before he eats. Sometimes even a fifteen-minute nap will help to settle your baby for a feed.

baby care tip

Eventually the night wakings to feed will phase out. If your baby wakes and only nurses for a few minutes, she probably wasn't really hungry. If this is happening, try not to feed your baby at night. As I mentioned, your baby will wake up during the night—we all do—but try to allow her to go back to sleep. If you consistently find that she is truly hungry and anxious to feed, try to feed her at 10 PM before you go to sleep by either waking her or, if possible, doing a dream feed while she's still sleeping.

There will be occasions when it is time for your baby to eat but he is not interested or simply refuses. Relax and do not let this worry you if it happens occasionally. Forcing your baby to eat and getting into a struggle is what you want to avoid. Your baby is telling you something by his actions. Has he had a very busy day? Has he napped enough? Sometimes babies of this age become irritable when they are overtired and stimulated. Try to put your baby down for a quick nap to refresh him. If he will not nap, try taking him for a walk in the stroller or in a sling or carrier. Eventually, when he is hungry, your baby will eat. It is OK if he misses a feed at this point. Believe me, he will make it up later.

Sleeping

· · · · · · · · · · · ·

At three months your baby will begin to sleep more soundly and have longer stretches of sleep—about five to eight hours during the night. If you are not seeing this five-hour stretch of uninterrupted sleep, you may need to establish some simple sleep routines. These routines will help your baby to learn how to fall asleep and stay asleep. Falling asleep is usually not the problem; staying asleep is. If your baby is able to get a solid stretch of sleep (some moms are happy with a three- or four-hour stretch), not only will you feel more rested, but your baby will also be much happier and content. Remember what we discussed about sleep at two months. When your baby wakes up or begins to whimper after only being asleep for a few hours, do not rush over to pick him up or feed him. Interfere as little as possible and try to allow your baby to fall asleep on his own.

Q. My baby is three months old and still not sleeping well during the night. We are up three to four times a night with her. Will moving her into her own room help?

A. Waking up several times during the night is normal sleeping behavior for a baby. The problem is that she cannot or does not know how to go back to sleep because she has not had the opportunity to learn. If you are not happy with your baby's current nighttime sleep habits, evaluate your current situation. As you consider whether to move her into her own room, remember the AAP's sleep guidelines that suggest baby share a room with parents until at least six months old.

In the meantime, you can help her learn to fall back to sleep by giving her some time. Do not rush to pick her up right away when you hear her fuss, and she will most likely go back to sleep within a short time. Some babies actually make quite a bit of noise during their light sleep stages, so your baby may not be fully awake. Try to give her ten or fifteen minutes before going over to her. I know this seems like a long time, but it may take that long for her to go back to sleep because she is not used to it. If her crying escalates and she is becoming very upset, go ahead and try to calm her down by rubbing her tummy and telling her that you love her. She may settle on her own in a few minutes. If your baby is too upset to settle down, pick her up and calm her. When she is calm but not asleep, put her back into the crib. Be consistent with this pattern over the course of a week and very soon you will have a baby who wakes up and goes right back to sleep.

baby care tip

Many babies will go through periods where they begin waking at night after they had been sleeping throughout. Often these wakings follow an illness or a disruption in routine such as a vacation away from home. Sudden nighttime wakening also may coincide with a new skill your baby is learning; for instance, she may be practicing to roll over, and once she does, she is stuck in this position and may wake herself up. When these wakings occur, try to stick with the routines that your baby is familiar with. Being consistent with your bedtime rituals will help to resolve this temporary problem.

Q. My baby's sleep seems to be regressing. He had been sleeping for eight to ten hours per night and now he wakes up at 4 AM and refuses to go back to sleep unless he's in my bed. Help! How can I get him back to his old sleep routine?

A. Babies will continue to surprise you: just when you thought they were sleeping through the night, they start to wake up again. This is a common problem that your baby will eventually (hopefully soon) outgrow. The fact that he falls asleep when he's in your bed means that he really is tired. He may like sleeping in your bed but you probably won't be able to get back to sleep (it's not safe). If this early morning waking continues, you may need to go back to the sleep training I discussed in chapter 11. When he wakes, do not take him out of the crib—let him fuss until he falls back to sleep. If you need to go pick him up, remember, do not rush over. If you give him enough time and he is not crying hysterically, he may fall asleep again.

Early morning waking tends to become a habit. It comes out of the blue and surprises parents who thought they had conquered the sleep battles. This is all OK as long as you follow the basic rules about getting him to go back to sleep.

Q. Does my baby still need regular daytime naps? Will he sleep better at night if I keep him awake during the day?

A. Your baby still needs daytime naps. In fact, napping during the day will help your baby to sleep better at night. Babies who are over-tired often have a hard time getting into a restful sleep state because adrenaline in their body takes over. So how long and how many naps should your baby have? Every baby is different—some take a few long naps during the day and others are catnappers taking several thirty- to forty-minute naps per day. If you have other children and your new baby is getting used to being on the go, he may have a catnap routine. There is nothing wrong with that as long as it's OK with you. Some parents prefer that their babies take fewer naps for longer periods of time. If this is something you would like for your baby, then it's best to try to stick to a sleep schedule—always keeping in mind the need for flexibility here and there. You can do this with a little planning ahead, to make sure you get home before you know your baby will get tired!

baby care tip

If you prefer that your baby take fewer naps but for longer periods, try to stick to a consistent napping routine. Pick a time of day when you will most likely be home. If you have older children, consider napping the baby after you drop them off at school in the morning. The baby can catnap for the rest of the day, but at least you can count on one regular nap time for a while.

Q. My baby sleeps fine at night—close to eight straight hours— but during the day she only sleeps for fifteen to thirty minutes at a time. She wakes up crying and still tired. What should I do?

A. First of all, is your baby falling asleep on her own unassisted? This is very important because this needs to happen if you want her to sleep for longer stretches. Most babies at this age need at least a sixty-minute nap to feel rested—and a rested baby is a happy baby! If your baby can get herself back to sleep on her own during the night, do not rush to her if she wakes twenty minutes after starting her nap. Let her fall back asleep on her own. You can set a timer (real or imaginary) and resolve not to take your baby out of the crib until an hour has passed. She will fuss for a while, maybe even the whole sixty minutes, but if you are consistent she will eventually begin to sleep longer.

It will be hard to hear your baby cry, so it's OK to go rub her back to calm her down. Remember, this does not mean you should put your baby in her crib to cry for an hour. You are still there to provide her with comfort and reassurance by rubbing her back and telling her that you love her in a calm voice. You will be surprised that within a few days your baby will fall back asleep after a few minutes. The key is being consistent, and understanding that you are helping her to learn a very valuable skill.

baby care tip

Sticking to a consistent schedule can be very helpful when you are trying to establish good sleeping habits for your baby. Of course, this cannot always be the case—you will occasionally have interruptions in the schedule for whatever reason. But overall, it helps to have some consistency in your day-to-day life.

Q. I'm all for my child establishing good sleep habits, but I don't like the idea of her "crying it out." It's not essential to do it that way, is it?

A. "Crying it out" is a controversial phrase that has many interpretations. Regardless of the interpretation, it's not essential to forming good sleep habits. Keep in mind that no one method works for everybody because all parents and babies are different. What feels right to one set of parents may not feel the same way for another. The same is true for babies—they are all born with different personalities and temperaments. I can't emphasize enough that the goal is to help your baby learn to fall asleep on her own. This is something that your baby needs and is capable of doing. Over the years, I have witnessed thousands of babies begin to sleep better once they've learned to fall asleep on their own.

Soothing

....

This section is nowhere near as detailed as the soothing sections in chapters 10 and 11 because your three-month-old will probably be a very happy little baby with big smiles and gurgles. Gone will be the days of constantly trying to keep her from crying and figuring out what tricks work best—she will now almost always have a reason when she cries. And aside from the basic reasons of hunger, a dirty or wet diaper, and fatigue, there may be a few new causes for your baby to be upset.

Teething

....

Some babies start teething at three months. If your baby starts drooling more significantly, putting his hands—or any object within his grasp—into his mouth, or all of a sudden rejecting the breast or bottle nipple while obviously hungry, a few teething-related crying spells may be in your near future. Often this can happen early, even when the teeth have not yet come close to the surface, which is why some parents don't pick up on the problem right away. If you do think your baby is upset because of teething, ask your pediatrician first if you're thinking about using anything to relieve pain or numb the gums. It's always best to try some of the following soothing methods first.

- Run a clean, soft, baby washcloth under cold water and wring it out. Put it in a plastic bag or container and store it in the freezer. Your baby may enjoy the feeling of the cold cloth between his gums.
- Put a soft plastic pacifier or teething ring in the freezer or fridge and allow your baby to gum on that.
- Wash your hands and gently but firmly rub back and forth on your baby's gums. Your baby will tell you whether or not the technique is working, and you can switch things up accordingly.

- While this may not address the teething pain directly, holding your baby close, rocking, and letting her hear the soft sound of your voice can be enough to calm her down and make her feel better.

In addition to teething, some cries can represent an ear infection, gassiness, or another sickness, so be on the lookout for signs of fever, ear pulling, or cold symptoms. Aside from these basic issues, your baby will be relatively easy to please at this stage. Of course, you will still have a baby and babies cry, but you will be able to settle him down once you figure out what he needs. And once you do, you will be amazed at how happy and smiley your baby becomes. It will seem that all of a sudden he is interested in everything around him, and you and the main caregivers in his life make him the happiest.

Development

In chapters 10 and 11 I mentioned the importance of talking to and reading with your baby—even at that early newborn stage of one and two months old. I want to emphasize the importance of making this kind of interaction a natural part of your day. And at three months old your baby will actually start to respond through movements, expressions, and sounds, making it more fun for you and creating an even more positive developmental experience for her. By regularly reading and communicating with your baby, you immerse her in language and ideas and build her knowledge of the world around her.

Consider this familiar family scene: A new mother prepares to take her baby girl out for a walk. She holds her infant lovingly, kisses her head while she puts on a tiny sweater, and explains aloud: "We need sweaters on today because it's cold outside and we're going for a walk!" As the mom is tying her baby's hat and placing her into the stroller, she elaborates, "Should we look for doggies out there today? Remember, we saw a big doggie yesterday! He was big and black and he liked to run after the ball. The doggie says, 'Woof, woof!' Let's go try and find the big black doggie!" It may be a little hard to believe, but it is critical to turn your everyday routines into an opportunity to talk to and interact with your baby in this way. The questions and explanations that this new mother consistently poses to her baby will ultimately be a major determinant in whether or not the baby becomes a strong reader, or perhaps even whether she goes on to graduate from high school.[39]

You might wonder why you should talk to your baby so much when she can't talk back at this point. But it turns out that the quantity and quality of language a baby hears from a parent greatly affects the child's vocabulary development.[40] And children's vocabulary growth is important; there is a well-documented link between strong oral vocabulary and strong reading skills. In fact, research shows that a child's vocabulary at age four predicts third-grade reading comprehension.[41] The kind of talk that goes on in your household and the conversations you have with your baby and with other family members make a difference. Studies show that parental speech should be both supportive (praising, asking questions) and complex (sophisticated vocabulary and ideas).[42] Since building strong language and thinking skills—both central to children's reading success—begins long before your baby can talk, you'll want to make certain that she lives in a language-rich environment.

If we return to our example, consider that before the pair have even taken one step outside, the baby has been exposed to more than fifty words and many different ideas that have been connected through speech. She has begun to learn about dogs and what noises they make and how they like to chase after balls, all while being tended to and cared for and spoken to in a loving way. In addition, while the mother may not notice it, she has used a complex sentence—she said that they need sweaters because it is cold outside. Over time, these kinds of sentences will help your baby learn how language works, and the causal relationship between the weather outside and wearing a sweater. In contrast, if the mother had simply kissed her baby's head and placed

---

39   C. E. Snow, M. D. Porche, P. O. Tabors, and S. R. Harris, *Is Literacy Enough? Pathways to Academic Success for Adolescents* (Baltimore: Brookes, 2007).

40   B. Hart and T. R. Risley, *Meaningful Differences in the Everyday Experience of Young American Children* (Baltimore: Brookes, 1995).

41   National Institute of Child Health and Human Development, *Teaching Children to Read: An Evidence-Based Assessment of the Scientific Research Literature on Reading and Its Implications for Reading Instruction: Report of the National Reading Panel.* NIH Publication No. 00-4769 (Washington D.C.: U.S. Government Printing Office, 2000).

42   Z. O. Weizman and C. E. Snow, "Lexical Input as Related to Children's Vocabulary Acquisition: Effects of Sophisticated Exposure and Support for Meaning," *Developmental Psychology* 37, no. 2 (2001): 265–79.

her lovingly in the stroller without conversation, the opportunity to build the baby's language and thinking skills would have been squandered.

baby care tip

How should you read to your baby? Just cuddle her in your arms, open the book, and enjoy! Some books you will want to read word for word, especially words with engaging rhythm, rhyme, or repetitive words. Others are better "read" by talking about the pictures and pointing out what is happening, reminding your baby when there are pictures of familiar things or people. Read and reread the books, day after day, and create a loving, warm, engaging, and language-rich experience that both you and your child will look forward to. As your baby begins teething and becomes more interested in *eating* the book, keep a chemical-free teether handy as you read.

When you elaborate for your baby, start with a loving and attentive manner and use basic words to communicate, and subsequently add more language and more ideas, you are working to expand your child's language and build her knowledge of the world. You are actually affecting her brain architecture because every new competency is built on competencies that came before.

But while talking to your baby and building up the number of words she hears is the first step, you also need to expose your child to the language of print, because written language is different from spoken language. Your baby will need to be familiar with the types of words and sentence constructions that are in books in order to be able to understand what she reads in the years to come. All of that learning should start early: Read to your baby and you'll cultivate a habit that will last a lifetime.

And remember, don't be afraid to use what seem like difficult words (the complex language that builds vocabulary and thinking skills), especially as you discuss the books you are reading together. Research shows that parents' use of sophisticated words, especially talk around books, predicts children's kindergarten and second grade vocabulary.[43] To support your child's understanding, take the time to

---

43   Weizman and Snow, "Lexical Input as Related to Children's Vocabulary Acquisition."

talk about and elaborate on what you read any time you are reminded of the book, too. Repeating the language will just continue to build up knowledge. So when that mother from our example sees that black dog again out on their walk, she might remind her baby of the dog in the famous children's book they read together:

"That black doggie looks just like Carl the dog![44] Do you remember we read about Carl the dog today? He took the baby for a ride on his back! How silly—babies shouldn't ride on dogs! We love Carl the dog, though, don't we?"

Establishing a habit early of reading with your baby will set up opportunities for practice with complex language now and in the years to come. We know that early reading ability predicts a child's success at middle school, and middle school success predicts high school academic achievement.[45] Entering kindergarten ready to learn can make all the difference—and all it takes is a decision by you to talk to and to read to your baby engagingly every day.

Stimulating Your Baby's Senses

Because your baby will no longer just be interested in sleeping and eating, he will be spending much more time watching and learning about the world around him—wanting to be part of the action! One of your most important jobs as a parent at this stage and onward is to help stimulate his senses in order to facilitate both intellectual learning and physical ability. Fortunately, this is both very easy and lots of fun. Here are a few suggestions on how best to engage your baby's senses.

Touch

During the first two months many babies like to keep their hands in tight fists, but at three months, suddenly your baby will notice that he has hands and will love to explore them. He will not only watch them

---

44   Alexandra Day, *Carl's Afternoon in the Park* (New York: Farrar, Straus & Giroux, 1991).

45   H. W. Catts, M. E. Fey, X. Zhang, et al., "Estimating the Risk of Future Reading Difficulties in Kindergarten Children: A Research-Based Model and Its Clinical Implementation," *Language, Speech, and Hearing Services in Schools* 32, no. 1 (2001): 38–50.

but will also start exploring his environment with them. He will likely be interested in holding toys and will probably bring anything he can up into his mouth. He may even notice his feet and toes, and will eventually be able to grab and bring those to his mouth, too. Take advantage of this development and give him toys—and simple, safe objects from around the house like measuring spoons—that have different shapes and textures. This will start to give him a sense of the many sizes, colors, and functions of the objects around him.

Hearing

Your baby will become much more vocal at three months. She will have her own baby language consisting of simple sounds such as "aaaaah." She may also gurgle, coo, or even slightly giggle when you play with her. All of these sounds indicate she is trying her best to communicate with you, so, as I emphasized earlier, talk to your baby as much as possible.

Here are some other great ways to engage your baby's hearing and overall development: Count, sing songs, name and describe the colors and textures of each toy she's playing with. When you show her books, point at the picture and name the object. Make different noises—for example, the cow goes "moo," the bee, "buzz," and so on.

Sight

Your baby will now become a lap baby—he'll be much happier when he is sitting up and able to watch the world around him. He will still need to be supported, but he'll hold his head up nice and strong. Sit him on your lap and show him some simple picture books, tapping on each picture to get his attention. Show him simple toys—move them around in front of his face so he follows them with his eyes. Roll a ball back and fourth, and up and down, and watch as he learns to follow it in different directions at various paces.

Because your baby will recognize your face and the faces of familiar people in his life, another way to stimulate him is through photographs. Walk around your home with your baby and point at photos on walls or flip through a photo album. As he learns that the faces in pictures are the same people who make him smile—and squeal with delight—in real life, his brain will make effective associations.

Taste and Smell

While there's really not much—as far as we know—you can do to improve your baby's senses of taste and smell, there's a lot you can do to stimulate and make associations with them. Here are a few ideas:

- When changing your dirty baby's diaper, hold your nose and react dramatically to the smell (which you may, in fact, do very naturally!). This will help your baby make an association from your nose to the sense of smell.

- When feeding your baby, ask him if his bottle or breast milk tastes yummy. This will help him make the association between taste and feeding.

baby care tip

If you are breastfeeding, try to eat many different types of foods to expose your baby to a variety of flavors. You may even notice that your baby protests at certain times or sucks differently depending on what you have eaten.[46]

Milestones

The list is getting much longer! By the end of the three-month period, your baby will have made the transition from a newborn to an active and responsive baby. At the end of this month your baby may:

- Raise the head and chest when on the stomach for tummy time
- Stretch the legs and kick when on the back or tummy
- Open and shut fingers
- Bring hands to the mouth
- Push down on legs when held in a standing position on your lap
- Try to bat or swipe at danging toys or objects
- Recognize and smile at you and other familiar people
- Begin to vocalize with cooing and babbling

---

46   N. Rones, "Your Baby's Developing Senses," *Parents*, parents.com/baby/development/physical/babies-developing-senses.

- Become more social
- Make expressive faces

> ### baby care tip
> The American Academy of Pediatrics recommends your baby be seen at birth, two to four days after birth, and at two months, four months, six months, nine months, and twelve months. There is no standard recommendation for a routine "well visit" at three months of age.

New Terrain for Mom: Work and Sex

Many moms return to work as their babies turn three months old. If you're one of them, be aware that although you may be excited to get back, you also may feel very emotional when the time comes. It can also be a challenge—not to mention expensive—to find quality child care, which can add anxiety. If you are not returning to work, finances might become stressful without that income, but on the plus side you save on child care and get to stay home with your little one! Other issues that typically arise around the three-month mark relate to your body image and sex. Just remember that all of these concerns are normal, and, with a little time, communication, and positive thinking, work themselves out rather seamlessly. I'll address some of the common concerns below and provide a suggested daily routine for the working mom.

Q. I'll be returning to work at the end of this month and I'm so anxious about leaving my baby in day care. Do all moms feel like this?

A. Yes—you are not alone. But I can tell you from having counseled hundreds of moms that the period leading up to your actual first day is the most stressful part. Of course, during the first few days of dropping your baby off, there might be a few tears—but usually only from you. At three months your baby will most likely be smiling, happy, and ready to interact with new faces. Of course he will miss you, but he is not likely to be old enough to experience separation anxiety, which at the earliest probably won't happen until about five months. When you pick your baby up at the end of your workday you will very likely have a smiling, happy child waiting for you. Thinking and worrying about leaving your baby will cause you a lot of anxiety. Even the most worried and teary moms tell me that returning to work was much easier than they had anticipated it would be. Most babies are very happy in their day care surroundings, and when you see this for yourself you will be happy as well. Try your best to relax, trust your child-care providers, and appreciate all of the social benefits your child will receive from spending his days among other children.

Choosing Child Care

Start by researching your child-care options while you are still pregnant—sometime in your third trimester. It will feel strange to think about this before your baby is even born, but in the long run it will be in everyone's best interest. (And in some areas of the country, early research and enrollment in day care centers is the only way you'll even get a spot in the one you want your baby to attend.) You'll want to explore several possibilities and in the end choose one that feels right for your family.

baby care tip

- Discuss your finances with your partner and know what you can and cannot afford.
- Discuss your child-care options with your partner—home day care, a day care center, or a babysitter/nanny—and decide which option you both feel is the best fit for your family's needs and schedule. It is important that you are both in agreement.
- Do your research and make a list of providers in your area.

Review your information and come up with a list of possibilities. Make appointments and visit each day care. Go with your gut feeling—if one doesn't feel right, cross it off of your list. If one is too expensive, cross it off your list. Make several visits to get familiar with the day care, including an unannounced visit so you can see how the day care operates when they are not expecting you. Once you have narrowed down your list, make another appointment to visit and find out how to secure a spot. After all your research is done, picture where or with whom you most trust your child and, again, go with your gut instinct.

baby care tip

When considering your child-care options, one of the best ways to find out about the quality of area day care centers or nannies is word of mouth. Post a question on your local family or mothers' group forum, asking if anyone has any recommendations or if they've had any good—or bad—experiences with a particular option you are considering. Chances are, if you hear several people respond with glowing reviews about a center you're considering, you'll feel confident in your selection.

QUESTIONS TO ASK YOUR PROSPECTIVE CHILD-CARE PROVIDERS

▶ **DAY CARE CENTER OR HOME DAY CARE**

- Is your day care licensed?
- What is the experience level and training process of your staff (pedagogical education, first aid, infant/child CPR–certified, etc.)?
- What is the infant-to-care-provider ratio?
- How much do you charge?
- What does the cost include?
- What are your visiting, dropoff, and pickup policies?
- What is a typical daily routine for infants?
- What kinds of activities and interaction will my baby be exposed to?
- Do you have a sick child policy?

▶ **NANNY OR BABYSITTER**

- What is your infant care experience level?
- Do you have past child-care employment references?
- What kinds of activities and interaction would you provide during the day?
- Do you have a clean driving record?
- Are you infant/child CPR–certified?

- Have you had any first aid training?
- Are your work hours flexible?
- What might you do if a baby was crying inconsolably for a long period of time?
- What is your hourly rate?

Q. My partner and I have decided to hire a nanny to care for our three-month-old in our home while we're at work. But I'm a little anxious about it because I'll be working full-time—what if my baby starts to think the nanny is her mom?

A. This is a common—but often secret—concern that moms have. But no matter if you have to work more than forty hours a week—your baby will know that you are her mom. Just make sure when you get home that your time is spent cuddling, talking, and playing with your baby instead of putting her straight to bed. Even if it's just for twenty minutes or a half hour, every minute of affectionate interaction counts. And if you start to feel guilty for being away or jealous of the nanny, remember that you decided to hire a nanny because the arrangement has huge benefits for your child. Having just a few main caregivers (parents and the nanny) will help your child build trusting relationships and confidence. And with one-on-one care, you'll know that your baby is receiving all of the attention to her safety and development that she deserves.

baby care tip

If you are set on hiring a nanny or babysitter and have extra money to put toward your search, consider hiring a local agency to help. Finding your nanny or babysitter this way can be pricey, but agencies pride themselves on finding only the best candidates. The nanny application process typically includes detailed child-care scenario essay questions and a personal interview, while references, child-care experience, a clean driving record, a CORI check, and infant/child CPR certification are often mandatory. You provide the company with your detailed needs and the salary range you can afford, and they'll send you candidates that match your family's needs.

Q. I've made the decision not to return to work. When should I let my employer know?

A. The sooner you do this, the better. It will not only give your employer time to find a replacement, but it will really be a weight off your shoulders once you share the news. Be sure to plan what you are going to say (or write, if it will be a formal resignation letter) before you do. Maintain a professional tone and thank them for the opportunities you've had working there—it never hurts to leave on a positive note with the door slightly left open in case things change somewhere along the line! Then you can relax and enjoy your time at home with your baby.

Q. I've made the decision to stay home full-time with my new baby. Financially it will be tough for us and I'm worried. Will I regret leaving my job?

A. This is a tough decision and you aren't alone in making it. It's normal to have some regrets cross your mind once in a while—the grass is always greener, after all! Concentrate on all of the benefits for your family that the decision to stay home brings. Perhaps you'll have to make cuts in spending here and there, but your baby will have the ultimate security (and that goes a long way) of having you there round the clock. The bond, sense of comfort, and memories the two of you create will stay with him throughout his life. Find local play groups and library story times where you can meet other stay-at-home parents, and make sure to allow for some truly free play and downtime every day. If things do get to a point where you really need to make some extra cash, do some research on ways you can work from home (freelance writing, sales jobs, or babysitting, for instance). If you are committed to finding something that suits your new lifestyle, you will.

Body Image and Sex

These days you may feel discouraged because your body no longer looks the way it did before pregnancy. It may be cliché, but it's true—it took nine months for your body to prepare for having a baby and it will take about that long for your body to return to its pre-pregnant state. If you do feel uncomfortable with your body, you may find that this contributes to an already decreased sex drive, so we'll address that below.

As we've discussed, exercise will make you look and feel better. Try to set some long-term fitness goals and start off with some basic cardio, yoga, or even just daily walks—anything that gets you moving.

Q. I'm still not fitting into my old clothes. Will my body ever look the same again?

A. Absolutely, there is no reason to think it will not, as long as you are taking care of yourself by eating healthy foods and getting some exercise every day. It is important not to think of your body as "long gone," but it will take some work and dedication to get back into those old clothes. The key is to take it day by day. If you got used to eating a certain not-so-healthy food (such as ice cream or frozen yogurt) during pregnancy, there's no need to eliminate it altogether. Just cut down your portion size, drink as much water as possible, and add more veggies during the day. Make it a priority for you and your baby to be active—take a walk or a light jog while pushing the stroller outside (or in the mall if the weather's bad). Wearing your baby on and off throughout the day in a carrier can also help you burn extra calories. Join a play group with moms who also have fitness goals to help motivate you to get out there and move. These are all healthy things you can do that your baby will benefit from and enjoy.

Q. When will my period return?

A. If you are not breastfeeding, your period will return sometime between three and ten weeks postpartum. If you are exclusively breastfeeding, the return of your period could be months away. It is important to understand that ovulation occurs before menses, so if you are sexually active with your partner you should use contraception, because you can get pregnant whether or not you are breastfeeding.

Q. I've lost interest in being physically intimate with my partner. Is this normal?

A. Yes—pregnancy and hormones tend to suppress your sex drive temporarily. I know it can be tough, and you may feel guilty because your partner wants to connect with you on a physical level. The number one reason you just aren't feeling it is fatigue (and you never know, he might be feeling the same way!). It can also be hard to feel intimate with your partner because you spend so much energy caring for your baby all day—and get plenty of cuddling along the way! By the time you're ready for bed, you may just want some time (or sleep) to yourself. But try to take advantage of this three-month mark because you will likely be sleeping a bit better. When you go to bed at night, make an effort to at least snuggle with your partner, which will help you start bringing some intimacy back. Lack of privacy can be an issue, so ask a friend or family member to stay with your baby for a few hours so you can go on a date with your partner. Just be sure to set aside some time to be romantic.

I can't emphasize enough how important it is that you talk to your partner about your feelings. You will connect with your sexual side again as your baby get older and less needy, but don't put pressure on yourself or your partner. You will still have days of being exhausted or overwhelmed, so take as much time as you feel you need.

Checking in with Dad (or Partner)

Dads/Partners, you may start to feel more of a bond with your baby at three months because at this point he can actually interact with you through smiles, cuddles, coos, and gurgles. When you read a book he will reach for it, and he will start to really observe the toys you play with together. If you sing the same songs regularly while you change his diaper, he will start to recognize them and show his excitement— perhaps by kicking his feet—upon hearing them. You, as a father, will also likely feel more confident in the day-to-day handling of your baby, and, best of all, you will finally know for sure that your baby recognizes you. Take advantage of all of these new developments and continue to interact with your baby in as many ways as possible. You will continue to see that bond between you and your baby grow in unique ways, and watching him reach his own daily developmental milestones will never cease to amaze you.

Q. My baby is definitely getting more interactive with me, but I still feel like there's not much we can do together. What kinds of things should we be doing at this stage?

A. Don't stress about what you "should" and shouldn't be doing. The absolute most important thing in your baby's life right now is building solid relationships with his parents through communication, interaction, and affection. As long as you provide these things, your baby will be on track developmentally and having lots of fun in the meantime! Here are a few simple ideas:

- Dress your baby in weather-appropriate clothing and go out for a walk. (You can do this in your own yard or head down the street, whatever works for you.) If possible, carry him in your arms or in a baby carrier. Especially if he is used to being carried primarily by another caregiver, it will be good for you two to have that closeness while he explores his environment. Describe various things you might see as you walk around—a red car, tall green trees, or white snow. Describe sounds he might hear—the birds chirping, a bus going by, or the wind blowing. You may think he won't understand you, but all of these interactions and associations will settle into his brain, and before you know it, you'll be shocked by all he does understand.

- Continue to read, read, read. Take the time to sit your baby on your lap as often as you can and read books. While it's good to have a few age-appropriate simple books to go through, there's nothing wrong with reading a few longer stories with big illustrations if your baby will sit through them happily. The sound of your voice will soothe him; he will get used to listening and paying attention, and will also continue to make valuable associations as you point to things in the book. Just be sure to read fairly slowly so he can hear each word clearly.

- Dance and sing with your baby. Put together a playlist of your favorite songs (nothing too harsh, of course) and designate it you and your baby's soundtrack. Every night when you get home, take your baby in your arms, put on your soundtrack, and dance and sing along. Your baby will love the closeness, the swaying motion, and hearing the different songs. He'll also learn to recognize this time as part of his routine, and will really look forward to it.

Q. It's been three months since our daughter was born and my wife and I still haven't had sex. I thought that after six weeks, when she was fully healed, things would go back to normal. Why haven't they?

A. Most women and even some men have a hard time returning to their sex lives after a new baby. The new schedule may leave your wife so tired that she just doesn't have the energy to even make the effort. Her hormones could also be affecting her physical sex drive so that she just may not have the desire. The best advice I can give—and that it will benefit you to take!—is to talk to your wife and be completely honest about your feelings. If you feel rejected, tell her that. But be sure to ask her how she feels, too. She may feel pressured or defensive if she feels you're blaming her for her decreased sex drive but will likely respond well if she feels you understand where she's coming from, so it's important to listen and truly try to consider her perspective. Sex and intimacy involves the two of you, so you need to be on the same page if you want to work toward a renewed sexual relationship that you're both happy with. Together, discuss different forms of intimacy you'd like to start with and how best to work them into your lives.

Suggested Daily Routines

If you are bottle-feeding, plan to give your baby five or six bottles each day containing five to six ounces of expressed breast milk or formula. If you are breastfeeding, your baby may need to feed at the breast more than six times a day.

Sample Routine for Working/Breastfeeding Mom and Working Dad with Twelve-Week-Old Baby

TIME	TASK	SUGGESTIONS
5:30 AM	Change/Breastfeed	Change your baby's diaper before the feed so that she's wide awake and gets what she needs. Burp after feeding.
6:00 AM	Sleep/Get ready for work	Swaddle your baby and allow her to go back to sleep while you pump remaining breast milk. You and Dad shower, eat breakfast, pack lunches (including expressed breast milk for child-care provider to feed baby), and pack clean pump and pumping supplies.
6:45 AM	Change/Play	When your baby wakes up, do not rush to feed her. Instead, sing and talk to her while you change her diaper. If you haven't already, pack lunches (including expressed breast milk for child-care provider) and pack clean pump and pumping supplies.
7:00 AM	Breastfeed	To help keep up your milk supply and give your baby a last quick feed, breastfeed for ten or so minutes if possible.
7:20 AM	Leave for child care/ Child-care provider arrives	Either pack up the car with essentials for the day at child care or, if you have someone come to your home, have your child-care provider come a little before you leave for work so you can give them an update and any necessary instructions.

TIME	TASK	SUGGESTIONS
7:50 AM	Dropoff/Leave	Drop your baby off with the child-care provider and/or leave for work.
8:00 AM–5:00 PM	Child care	Child-care provider feeds and takes care of the baby according to your recommendations. You receive a report of your baby's day when you pick her up. She will drink three or so bottles during the day.
5:30 PM	Play	Hold, cuddle, and sing to your baby. Sneak in a few minutes of face-to-face tummy time.
6:00 PM	Breastfeed/Prepare dinner	While you breastfeed and burp your baby, Dad can unpack your bags, wash the used bottles, pumping supplies, bibs and/or clothes, and ideally prepare dinner.
6:30 PM	Play/Dinner	Put your baby in a place where she can see you, and continue talking and interacting while you eat dinner.
7:00 PM	Bath/Massage	Together, give your baby either a calm bath or a massage with lotion to get her relaxed and ready for bed.
7:15 PM	Change	Gently sing to your baby as you change her diaper. Get her dressed for bed and read a story.
7:30 PM	Breastfeed	Sit in the rocker and breastfeed. Burp lightly.

TIME	TASK	SUGGESTIONS
8:15 PM	Sleep	Swaddle your baby, put her in the crib still awake, close the door, and listen on the monitor.
8:30 PM	Downtime	Take this time to clean up from dinner, make the next day's lunch, iron your clothes for work, and catch up on e-mail or other household tasks.
11:30 PM	Change/Breastfeed/Sleep	Depending on how much your baby receives during the day, she may be hungry one more time before her longer stretch of sleep. This can be a good time to do a "dream feed" and put her back down to sleep.
4:15 AM	Change/Breastfeed/Sleep	If your baby wakes up early in the morning, bring her into bed for a feeding, then swaddle and return her to her crib to catch some more sleep before the day begins.

At this point in your baby's life, your family will find a routine that works for all of you. Yes, there may still be the occasional midnight wakeup or day where your little one is extremely fussy and you don't know why. But with a little practice and the experience of having gotten to know your baby over three months, things will not only get smoother, but they'll start to get a lot more fun. Every day for the rest of your baby's first year will be filled with excitement as you wonder just what new noise or physical ability he will master next! Enjoy every moment of it (even those low-on-sleep, high-on-frustration days) and capture some of this time, whether in a baby book, photos, or film, because it'll all go by so fast. Before you know it, you'll treasure looking back on your baby's innocent newborn stage.

· 13 ·

....

From Newborn
to Toddler:
Bring on the Milestones!

....

After your newborn's first three months, you will begin to see
your baby's development and growth start to blossom. While
your baby may already have reached milestones by this time, such as
the first smile or rolling over, by the end of the year he will have met
dozens of them. Your baby will find his feet, sit up, get his first teeth,
gain complete control of his hands, eat solid foods, and the list goes
on and on. Although you may glance back and wonder where all of the
time has gone, and slightly miss the newborn stage, every day will get
better and better because your baby will continue to gain skills and
increase the fun interactions between you.

As a baby nurse and lactation consultant, I find that the families
I work with really start to get into a rhythm around this time. Even
those families who have gone through trials with breastfeeding, infant
sickness, or long-lasting colic tend to start seeing a difference in their
baby—feeding and sleeping become routine, and their babies' personalities start to shine through as they happily communicate. There's a
lot you can take advantage of when your baby reaches this slightly
more independent stage. Here's a glance at the rest of your baby's
year.

Four to Six Months

· · · · · · · · · · · · ·

Eating

- Your baby will need regular bottle- or breastfeeding sessions throughout the day.

- Before starting your baby on solids, discuss a strategic introduction of various foods with your baby's pediatrician. This will help ensure you're providing your baby with optimal nutrition *and* taking steps to identify any potential food allergies. In 2015, the AAP highlighted that introducing peanuts earlier on may reduce the risk of a potentially life-threatening allergy in high-risk populations.[47]

- If you are interested in making your baby's food, simply buy a small food mill (there are some great ones for around just $10). Food mills are easy to use, easy to transport, and easy to clean. They also make perfectly sized portions for your baby. Make sure to wash all produce with cold water for thirty seconds.

- Good starter fruits and veggies are avocados, apples, bananas, peas, carrots, and sweet potatoes. You can also buy packaged baby food (both conventional and organic baby food are available at most grocery stores); look for "Stage 1" on the label, as it provides a smooth texture.

- Once your baby begins solid foods you will notice an immediate change in stool color, texture, and scent, particularly if your baby is breastfed and typically has loose stools. They will now be thicker, typically the color of the foods eaten, and have a stronger odor.

---

47 American Academy of Pediatrics, "AAP Joins in Interim Guidance on Introduction of Peanuts for High Risk Infants," press release, August 31, 2015, aap.org/en-us/about-the-aap/aap-press-room/pages/AAP-Joins-in-Interim-Guidance-on-Introduction-of-Peanuts-for-High-Risk-Infants.aspx.

> ## baby care tip
> Apples, bananas, and carrots can be constipating, so if you notice that your baby has not had a dirty diaper in a few days, you may want to take a break from those foods. Giving your baby fibrous fruits such as prunes can help move the digestion along.

Sleeping

- Your baby will likely still be taking naps every three hours (unless he is in a structured environment, such as day care, where he will likely only take two). This is a good time to institute a regular nap schedule; you can even try to consolidate your baby's sleeping into two long daytime naps. A good time for these naps would be morning from about 9 AM to 11 AM and in the afternoon around 2 PM to 4 PM.

- It is possible that your baby may still not be sleeping through the night at this point (or did so initially but has regressed to waking), which can be frustrating. Stick with the sleep tips I provided in chapters 11 and 12 and your baby will eventually get into a good sleeping routine. Even if some not-so-good sleep habits have formed in the first few months, it is possible to sleep train. It takes time and commitment (and some long nights!), but everyone will be better off in the short and long term.

Development

- Read books. At this stage your baby will be able to hold the books you read and even start to turn the pages on his own. (You'll find that the pages will be turned long before you get a chance to finish reading the text on the page!) This quality time bonding with your child is key, and the absorption of language is crucial.

- Take walks to the park. At this point your baby will be able to sit in the bucket swings, and she'll love being outdoors and around other kids.

Milestones

At this point your baby may:

- Roll over
- Steadily grasp objects
- Eat some solid foods (Stage 1 if storebought)

Seven to Nine Months

. . . .

Eating

- Your baby will need bottle- or breastfeedings when he wakes and goes to bed as well as throughout the day.
- Chances are your baby will be ready to advance to foods with a little more texture, so if you're buying baby food, look for "Stage 2" options. If you're making baby food, feel free to add a few mild spices and herbs. You can start to introduce meats, mild cheese, and pasta around this time, but always make sure that anything you serve to your baby is sliced into very small pieces that your baby can manage easily with bare gums.
- You can introduce a sippy cup with breast milk or formula at mealtimes, and fill it with water when out and about.

Sleeping

- Your baby will likely be taking two regular naps per day, each about two hours in length.
- Your baby should be sleeping through the night, going to bed sometime around 7 PM and waking sometime around 7 AM.

Development

- Consider enrolling in a baby music class. The structured yet creative environment among your baby's peers will help your baby learn about social interaction, listening, rhythm, and much more.

- Take your baby to your local library for a baby story time to foster his love for reading and learning about his environment.
- This is the time when your baby is likely to have some degree of separation or stranger anxiety.

Milestones

At this point your baby may:

- Sit without support
- Crawl (close to nine months)
- Pull self up
- Pass objects from hand to hand
- Object when you take a toy away
- Say "ma ma" or "da da" (closer to nine months)
- Play peekaboo
- Stand alone for a second (at least nine months)
- Cruise furniture: stand and "walk" while holding onto furniture for support (at least nine months)
- Respond to name when spoken to (around nine months)
- Grab a spoon during mealtime, and turn head when finished eating (nine months)
- Make sounds, razzing and imitating adult noises

baby care tip

Introduce healthy eating habits from the start. Your baby will get all the nutrition he needs through the fruits, veggies, and breast milk or formula you provide. During his first year particularly, avoid introducing sugary items such as fruit juice, cookies, cake, soda, and ice cream. Also refrain from giving him high-sodium things like chips or cheese-flavored crackers.

Ten to Twelve Months

· · · · · · · · · · · ·

Eating

- Your baby will need bottle- or breastfeedings when she wakes and goes to bed as well as throughout the day.
- Be prepared to share—at this stage your baby will want to eat everything you're eating. This can work to your advantage, though, especially if she starts refusing to eat during some of her mealtimes. The novelty of receiving something from your plate, even if it's the same thing that's on hers, may help her take enough nutrition. Simply cut up the food on your plate into tiny pieces and put it onto hers.
- Of course, getting your baby to eat everything that is offered to her won't always be so easy. Just remember to look at the big picture—as long as she eats a wide variety of fruits, veggies, and whole grains throughout the week, there's no need to battle to the death just because she won't eat her peas one night.

Sleeping

- By this time your baby's sleep routines should be relatively solid. She may cry out when you put her to bed (because there's so much to see and learn now!), but she also may be at a point where she knows when she's tired and enjoys her naps and sleep time.
- There will inevitably be some days where your baby doesn't sleep her full nap time or wakes up far too early in the morning. This is normal, so don't allow all of your hard work on her sleep routines to go out the window! If your baby does wake up early or just won't sleep during a regular nap time, make sure you leave her in her crib for at least a half hour. She may not sleep, but at least she'll be resting, and it's important that she have this downtime.

Development

- Continue to expose your baby to structured environments regularly, such as story time at the library or music class to encourage listening and social skills.
- Continue to read with your baby every day. It's a valuable part of language development, fosters a love of reading, and bonds the two of you.
- Separation anxiety can peak around this time, so transitions to another caregiver can pose a challenge. Always remember to say goodbye, as opposed to just "disappearing." Your baby will learn that you always come back and the anxiety will eventually subside.

Milestones

At this point your baby may:

- Have a few first words. Whether or not this happens, your baby will likely be very efficient at communicating her needs to you. But for those times when you don't know what she wants, be prepared for signs of a tantrum—it can be frustrating for her not to have enough words for all that she wants to do, eat, and see!
- Crawl very well
- Stand alone or take first steps
- Roll a ball back to you
- Respond to one-step commands

You have so many moments to look forward to as an expectant parent. By going through these pages filled with the experiences of so many new moms and dads—and the health-care providers who've guided them—you have equipped yourself with the knowledge you need to enjoy the labor and birth of your baby, each sweet (and sometimes sour) moment with your newborn, and every milestone in the coming year as your baby grows. As I have detailed, being a parent will be challenging at times. From the day my first child was born—until this year when I dropped him off at college—I have felt those challenges. Once you feel you've mastered the art of soothing your baby, establishing a successful bedtime routine, or getting him to eat his veggies, there will be yet another parenthood puzzle to solve. Just know that the joy you'll feel in forming a bond with and taking care of your baby makes it all worth it—the thousands of new moms I've worked with are a solid testament to that! Yes, there's a lot to think about as you prepare for this new venture in your life, but just turn to your support network and health-care provider, as well as baby-related resources (this book!), when you need a little guidance.

Appendix

For more information on sudden infant death syndrome (SIDS), contact:

American SIDS Institute

Nonprofit providing SIDS research, education, and family support.
(239) 431-5425
sids.org

CJ First Candle

Provides education, training, advocacy, and bereavement services, including a twenty-four-hour bereavement counseling helpline in English and Spanish.
(800) 221-7437
cjfirstcandle.org

National Sudden and Unexpected Infant/Child Death and Pregnancy Loss Project IMPACT

Serves as the communications hub for a national network of fetal, infant, and child mortality programs—convening, connecting, and providing technical support to state and local efforts.
(800) 930-7437
sidsprojectimpact.com

National Sudden and Unexpected Infant/Child Death and Pregnancy Loss Project at the National Center for Cultural Competence

Provides technical assistance and develops resources on cultural and linguistic competence to help programs effectively address racial and ethnic disparities in perinatal, infant, and child mortality and pregnancy loss.
(800) 788–2066
E-mail: cultural@georgetown.edu
nccc.georgetown.edu/projects/sids

Safe to Sleep Campaign: Eunice Kennedy Shriver National Institute of Child Health and Human Development

(800) 505–2742
E-mail: nichdinformationresourcecenter@mail.nih.gov
nichd.nih.gov/sids

Acknowledgments

In addition to raising my three children, writing *Newborn 101* has been one of my greatest and most rewarding challenges. I could not have done it without the help of many talented individuals. I extend my sincere gratitude to them all. I feel lucky to have been surrounded by such a supportive group of experts.

Thank you to my friends who contributed their unique skills and knowledge as my unofficial editors, medical advisors, and support team: Thanks to Dr. Paula McEvoy for reviewing my manuscript and sharing her expertise about newborns. Her friendship and professional collaboration mean a great deal to me. My heartfelt thanks to Dr. Carrie Stucken for offering her generosity, time, and medical wisdom, and for writing such a wonderful testimonial. Thanks to Abbey Tiderman—a wonderful friend and editor—for proofreading and helping me develop the manuscript. Abbey's editing skills combined with her hands-on experience raising two young boys made her perfect for the job. I couldn't have done it without her.

Thank you to Joëlle Delbourgo, my agent, for believing in my work and helping me achieve my goals. Thank you to Matthew Lore and the team at The Experiment. Thank you to Batya Rosenblum, for her expert editorial guidance. Thanks to Diana Herman for being my constant support and right hand, Danica Cheslofska for being the creative force behind Boston Baby Nurse, Erica Ruggles for keeping my schedule organized and for her great social media posts, Katie Zereski, founder of Yummy for Mommy, for her valued breast feeding expertise, Diane Lopes for her experience as an educator and sleep coach, as well as the entire team of overnight Newborn Care Specialists. Thanks to my friends who have given me the encouragement and support I've needed over the past few years.

Above all, thank you to my family for being so supportive and helpful and for always being willing to give me the time I needed to write and complete this book. Thank you to Marc, Michelle, Doreen, and my three children, Alex, Cam, and Caroline, for being so accepting of my preoccupation with *Newborn 101* over the last few years. Special thanks to my brother Tom, sister-in-law Corinne, and my niece and nephew—Emmy and Pete—who I've had the privilege of spending time with since they were newborns. And a big thank-you to my mom and dad, Ingrid and Gunter Kramer, for being so understanding and for always believing in me! I look forward to spending more time with all of you now that the book is complete.

Index

About the Author

CAROLE KRAMER ARSENAULT, RN, IBCLC, is a nurse, parent educator, certified lactation consultant, and the founder of Boston Baby Nurses, Boston's leading baby nurse company. Arsenault and her ever-growing team of nurses have helped hundreds of parents through pregnancy, labor, birth, and the transition to their new role as caregivers with advice on breastfeeding, soothing, baby-care products, sleep schedules, and infant development. Arsenault and her team also provide lactation consulting to clients at Boston's top birthing hospitals, including Brigham and Women's Hospital, Beth Israel Hospital, St. Elizabeth's Medical Center, Newton-Wellesley Hospital, Massachusetts General Hospital, and Mount Auburn Hospital.

Arsenault practiced as a labor and delivery nurse at Brigham and Women's Hospital for many years, and is also an expert on environmental toxins that may affect pregnant women and newborns. Arsenault has been interviewed on common baby-care mistakes by Fox News online and is a monthly contributor to digital resources including *Boston Mamas* and the *Bump*. She lives near Boston with her husband and their three children.